O9-BTL-468

Don't Walk Through the Mirror

by *Anthony J. Garbowski*
& Lorna J. Shaw

© Copyright 2007, Anthony J. Garbowski & Lorna J. Shaw
Photographs & Cover Design by Lorna J. Shaw

All rights reserved. No part of this book may be reproduced or transmitted in any form or by any means, electronic or mechanical, including photocopying, recording, or by any information storage and retrieval system, without permission in writing from the publisher/authors.

The ideas and suggestions in this book are not intended to substitute for the help and service of a trained professional. All matters regarding your health require medical consultation and supervision. Always consult your doctor, lawyer and other professionals. All doctors' names in this book are fictional.

McMillen
Publishing.
A Sigler Company

Library of Congress Control Number: 2005932532
ISBN: 1-888223-70-7

1. Male Caregivers 2. Breast Cancer 3. Chronic Illness
4. Male Single Parents 5. Grieving

Anthony J. Garbowski has also authored *Profiting For People, By People*, a business book written in the corporate storytelling mode.

**Please feel free to
email the authors at
dontwalkthroughthemirror@yahoo.com**

DEDICATION

This book is dedicated in loving memory of Nancy Garbowski
&
John and Phyllis Shaw.

Don't Walk Through the Mirror

"I dreamed I was looking at my reflection in a mirror. I walked through the mirror and saw that on one side I was alive and on the other side I was dead. I remember calling out to you, Anthony, not to walk through the mirror or you will be dead like me."

My wife, Nancy, had wakened me in the dark, in the middle of the night. She told me about her terrible nightmare. It was about one year before she was to die. It was a stage in our lives when there were times I could feel death looking in our windows. In our bedroom, we had a chest of drawers with two large mirrors hanging above it.

Nancy's dream reflected her realization that her cancer was spreading and death was not only inevitable but near. When she finally did pass through the mirror, she left me behind with instructions to live and love again.

Little did I know, that nightmarish evening, how many mornings I would awaken after Nancy's death with a hard knot of anxiety in the pit of my stomach. On such mornings, the pain of loss and self-pity would be so great that I would often feel I would be better dead than alive. The mirrors were right there in my bedroom, beckoning me.

Since she died, I am much more aware of the impact that chronic, serious illnesses, and death of a loved one, have on people who are in close, loving relationships. Many times, when an elderly person dies, it is not long before the spouse passes away, walking through the mirror, following in the footsteps of their dearly beloved.

The purpose of this book is to share my insights with you in the hope of helping you cope successfully and with empathy with your loved one's illness. May it also give you the strength to heed Nancy's admonition:

DON'T WALK THROUGH THE MIRROR!

Acknowledgements

First we want to thank *Margaux Garbowski-Jacks*, for sharing so many of your daughter-mother recollections and in particular for allowing us to photograph your original painting, entitled, Pocahontas.

Heartfelt thanks also go to *Michelle Koch*, for your undying enthusiasm from the very beginning to the very end of our ten year labor of love. Bless you for "believing" and for your most insightful guidance and suggestions!

Sincerest thanks too, to *Joe Carbo*. Your past, present and future hands-on computer expertise has been priceless, as has your wholehearted backing and encouragement.

We cannot thank *Betty Dyck* enough for so eagerly assisting us with editing suggestions during both the earlier and later phases of *Don't Walk Through the Mirror*.

Nick Lemieur, we greatly appreciate your so cheerfully sharing your precious time and technical knowledge with us.

We are also grateful to *Aileen* and *Murray Shaw*, *Maureen* and *Doug Koch*, *Ted Cowan* and *Dennis Matthews*, for taking the time to read our earliest galley proofs and also for your thoughtful comments on our "work in progress."

Last, but certainly not least, we most sincerely thank *Jean Sachs, Bob Priem, Linda Welsh, Sandra Timmins* and *Elizabeth Monaghan*, for your tangible encouragement and support.

And in closing, author to author.........
Tony, how can I ever thank you enough for inviting me

into your most private world of feelings? How can I, on behalf of all the readers of *Don't Walk Through the Mirror*, thank you enough for sharing such intimate insights into the male psyche? After spending sixteen years on an emotional roller coaster alongside Nancy, you spent an additional ten years on an emotional roller coaster with me, so that those experiencing similar challenges involving chronic illnesses, can hopefully feel much less intimidated. WE THANK YOU!!

Lorna, I wish to acknowledge your incredible dedication to our book. For years, working under extremely challenging conditions, you devoted countless hours and exercised extreme patience transforming the focus of our work from Nancy's story to my experiences and feelings while supporting her. Thanks too for your helpful personal insights, resulting from several lengthy caregiving experiences of your own, which are intimately woven into the text. You also created a hauntingly mystical cover and enriched our text with marvelous illustrations. When bouts of grieving made it too difficult for me to go on, there were many times you carried the torch single-handedly. Everyone who benefits from this book is deeply indebted to you.

CONTENTS

Chapter 4 **Recurrence**

While recurrence is not a death-sentence, it is a traumatic milestone. How will you deal effectively with the psychology of recurrence and the debilitating effects of treatment? What new challenges will you encounter and what new demands will be made on you? Where can you muster up help and support?

Old feelings combine with intense new feelings. Hope can change to despair, anguish and anxiety. You may feel very discouraged when, in spite of all the treatments, hard work and sacrifice, cancer strikes again.

Chapter 5 **Intense stages**

Are you ready for the battle of your life? It will feel as if your life is in the balance along with that of your loved one. As the cancer spreads, treatments intensify with higher risks of side effects. New dangers may emerge as cancer invades new organs, bones and tissues. Your loved one may even be robbed of the ability to do the simplest things. How do you keep yourself physically and mentally strong during this highly stressful time?

Chapter 6 **Final stages**

Until recent years, seriously ill patients would often die in a hospital. Now, with cost containment, terminally ill cancer patients are sent home or to intermediate care facilities. What are your options? What are the advantages and disadvantages? What is hospice and is it for you? How can you find dependable home nursing care and what are the financial implications? While you will hear talk of a patient's rights, there are no laws or rules acknowledging and respecting the care provider's rights. You need to do this for yourself.

As your loved one approaches death, unless previous funeral arrangements have been made, you may have some very difficult decisions to make, such as selecting urns or caskets and deciding upon inground burial or cremation or mausoleums.

The Story of the Statue

Chapter 7 **Grieving**
If death becomes imminent, some people commence the grieving process before their loved one dies. Others postpone grieving, clinging to the hope that the patient will make yet another comeback. This chapter helps you understand what to expect, how to find support, and the impact on the rest of your life.

Chapter 8 **Their Spirit Lives On**
There is an aspect of death that cannot be seen, touched or quantified. After your loved one has died, you might experience extrasensory perceptions. What might these be? What do they signify?

Chapter 9 **Life Goes On**
While life does go on, you may find yourself challenged in ways you cannot foresee or fully comprehend. Many individuals will work their way through to new life. However, if you are now a single parent, be prepared to be patient and gentle with yourself, and with your children.

Chapter 10 **New Life**
This phase is both difficult and exciting, unwanted and desirable. Do you feel you want or deserve a new life? This chapter explores the transformation which can result from the grieving process. How do you get back into the social swing of things? How should the attitudes and expectations of your children, family and friends be handled? What does it mean to be a single parent and how does the parent's and the child's grieving process differ?

To Each His Own
An unknown author's advice

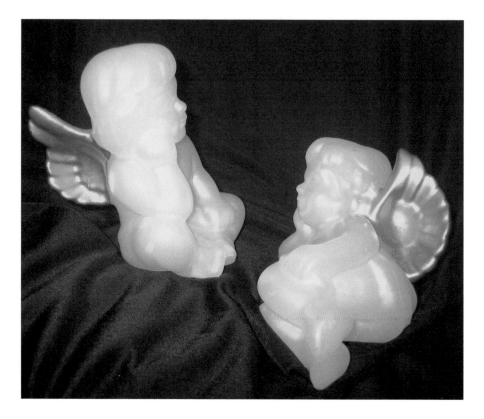

*Time will fly
and so will I!
We will be together again.*

INTRODUCTION

"I hold that a person of worth, who is in love, ought to be sincere and truthful in this as in all other things. I believe that gentle lovers endure so many toils, so many vigils, and are exposed to so many dangers, shed so many tears, use so many ways and means to please their love—not chiefly in order to possess the body, but to take the fortress of the mind. This I believe is the true and sound pleasure and the goal aimed at by every noble heart." (Adapted from Castiglione's *The Courtier*)

These words were written over 450 years ago. The concept was refined by the Renaissance poets, Dante and Petrarch. The philosophical idea of "gentility" can help you today when a loved one is confronted with a diagnosis of cancer, Alzheimer's or any serious or incurable illness. This concept encourages you to keep love in the relationship and to maintain a balance between the needs of the body and of the mind.

This Renaissance notion of love also emphasizes there is more to love than intimacy, more than the physical. Watching a loved one die can be an extremely spiritual experience.

It's okay to cry. Suppressing your emotions will only make it more difficult for you to get through the stresses and strains of any chronic illness. It will also hinder your ability to process and move forward when it is time to start a new life.

Cancer can be a relentless disease. In her last years Nancy referred to it as a "stalker." It was always there in some form, afflicting the mind and spirit as well as the body. To me, it felt like a roller-coaster ride that would not end. It was a constant series of highs and lows. The victories were exhilarating. Then, inevitably, there were the devastating losses. It was as if I were always on a tightrope, high above the ground, never being allowed to relax or drop my guard without serious consequences. At the time, I was, for the most part, unaware of how much this was draining me both physically and emotionally. Looking back, I now realize I had imperceptibly grown accustomed to living with a constant undercurrent of tension, stress and uneasiness. The fear of cancer had permanently infiltrated our life experiences.

Cancer has a tremendous impact on the entire family unit. As men sometimes have difficulty connecting with their feelings and often do not publicly express how they feel, such issues significantly affect the support a woman with breast cancer receives from the most important person in her life.

Nancy would come home from a support group meeting and talk about husbands who had left their wives. I found it incomprehensible that the partner in a caring, loving relationship would react to any disease in such a manner. Do we truly understand enough about how male caregivers are impacted? The patient receives the bulk of the attention and available medical resources, including counseling. Do husbands or partners have special significant needs that are not being addressed? I hope to answer some of these questions by writing this book from a man's point of view.

Children also feel threatened by the disease. They fear losing a parent. Looking back, putting myself in my daughter's shoes, I now realize that our daughter, Margaux, lived every day of her growing up years thinking she might lose her mom at any moment. This reality intensified when Nancy was bedridden in the nursing home. Margaux would visit on the weekends, and go back to school, thinking that each time could possibly be the last time she would see her mother alive.

How vividly I remember Margaux's lashing out at me shortly after her mother died, "You can find another spouse, but I lost the only mother I will ever have." It's not surprising children can act out feelings of anger, hurt and abandonment at this stage. And, at this time, it is the grieving man, totally unaccustomed to the role of single parent, who must step out of his own pain and loss to help surviving children.

The purpose of this book is to bring such issues to the surface, and it is our hope, in some small way, to improve one's understanding and ability to cope with the dynamics of any chronic life-threatening illness.

Additionally, this book provides much needed emotional and psychological support for male caregivers. In turn, the multitude of women dealing with cancer and chronic diseases will benefit from stronger, more empathetic male support providers.

First, there's an overview of our medical journey. I'm sharing this with you, up front, to give you a road map of the direction a life-threatening, incurable illness may take. Keep in mind, every person's experience is individual. Certainly, not everything that happened to us will happen to you. Many individuals never experience recurrence. Each disease works in its own unique way. However, the broad strokes of this story will be repeated many times over until cures are found.

Ironically, in my case, when my wife, Nancy, was first diagnosed with breast cancer, a disquieting memory from our past flashed through my mind. It occurred during my first opera, of many, with Nancy, which involved Franco Corelli and Renata Tebaldi in Puccini's *La Boheme*. I had never been to an opera before and I had difficulty understanding what was going on. I was not even sure I liked it as it was so different from anything I had ever experienced. The ending had had a profound effect on me. Disquieting. When Mimi died I had a premonition that Nancy would also die before me. Somehow, like poor Rodolfo, I would watch her die. It was silly. We had just met a few weeks before. We were just dating. The thought of marriage had not even entered the relationship. Not only was it silly to entertain such feelings, the feelings were disturbing and I put them out of my mind.......until now.

Here we were not only facing Nancy's mortality straight on, but also immediate prospects of a modified radical mastectomy. It was a sudden and significant transition for both of us to come to grips with Nancy's not having one breast.

Soon after her mastectomy, we were informed that the cancer had spread to lymph nodes under her left arm. Nancy was offered radiation and chemotherapy. She tried chemotherapy and elected not to continue this treatment because of its debilitating side effects. At that time, to refuse treatment was viewed as a very radical decision. From the outset Nancy was concerned about the quality of her life.

By taking time to become informed about her condition and the treatments, Nancy took control. She would often say it was her life and her body and no one had the right to dictate treatments to her. However, managing her illness in this manner put pressure on me. When she considered working outside accepted practices, I, in turn, felt a tremendous responsibility to support her through this major decision. Additionally, deep down, her decisive action increased my fears that she might die much sooner, robbing us of time together and leaving me alone to take care of our child on my own.

Fortunately, after the first surgery, Nancy experienced almost seven years without recurrence. At that time, doctors congratulated her, citing statistics that most patients, who survived for five years, would be free of cancer for the rest of their lives. I felt a huge sense of relief and hoped that we would now be able to lead a regular life. However, about seven years after her first surgery, our hopes were dashed when her cancer came back in the form of a nodule along the old surgical line, which necessitated a second operation.

About two years later, she had surgery to remove another tumor in the same area. A year or two after that, a third nodule had penetrated the muscles of the chest wall. Unfortunately, this tumor had lodged itself under the clavicle. Her surgeon therefore recommended an aggressive course of radiation therapy.

The cancer then spread to the bones of her spine, necessitating another major course of radiation. Each surgery, each major radiation treatment, placed increasing responsibilities on my shoulders. Not only did I help her process her innermost feelings and make decisions, I struggled with my own emotions. It seemed as if my life were completely out of control.

Then, fourteen years after the initial signs of cancer, Nancy started to experience memory loss. At first it was barely noticeable. Gradually, I observed she would stop in mid-sentence, forgetting what she wanted to say. A CAT scan of the head indicated she now had a brain tumor. Additional tests were performed and several small liver tumors were also discovered. Her radiation oncologist told me, "If it were anyone else walking into my office off the street, I would say she had 3-4 months to live."

I still remember that cold damp January day when they took Nancy in to 'map' and measure her radiation fields. I went for a slow, long walk down the hill behind the hospital. Crying in the freezing air, I was in shock. I felt sad, scared and sorry for myself.

Shortly thereafter, Nancy had major radiation to the head, accompanied by massive doses of steroids to reduce swelling of the brain tumor, thereby relieving the danger of pressure to the brain. The plan was then to commence aggressive chemotherapy during which she suffered the indignity of losing her hair.

In a matter of weeks, the treatments almost killed her. She became so weak she could not stand. Nor could she go unassisted to the bathroom. Besides severe memory loss, she expressed huge amounts of unresolved anger.

I did not like being the object of her anger and her frustrations during her illness and I often felt overwhelmed taking care of her. Over and over I placed my needs second to hers and suffered debilitating lower back pain when I helped her get up and go to the bathroom.

Her weakness led to two and a half months of shuttling back and forth between nursing homes and hospitals. During this entire time she was unable to come home and she required several blood transfusions which necessitated a surgically installed port.

The pressures on me seemed unbearable as I felt an inner need to visit her at the nursing home several times a day, while also keeping my job and caring for the house. Then too, it was my job to encourage Margaux, our daughter, to go back to college each Sunday afternoon after her weekend visits. I had to tell her that everything was under control and that she could help most by going back to school and by getting good grades. In actual fact, deep inside, I felt like I was drowning and part of me was screaming, "Help Margaux. Please stay and help us!" However, Margaux was already completely giving up her social life and free time at university so she could come home every weekend to help and be with her mother. Besides, her mother would not tolerate even the mention of Margaux's dropping out of school for a semester.

Miraculously, Nancy came home that spring. Incredibly, she commenced chemotherapy and tolerated cytoxine and 5 f-u well. I wanted to accompany her to as many treatments as possible. Due to her memory loss, I was the note taker and custodian of her long list of questions. Between treatments, she would depend on me to serve as her memory of what had been discussed. All this came on top of rapidly intensifying requirements and demands on the job. Juggling schedules to get my work done, and also being there for Nancy, became a staggering proposition.

Then, around the winter break holidays, her oncologist wanted her to have a rest from treatment. However, within a week or two, Nancy noticed several little pimples on her left chest. They itched and bothered her. I told her not to scratch or squeeze. In a matter of weeks this cancer recurrence turned into a two inch by four inch mass of white, yellow and red necrotic tissue.

Chemotherapy was hastily resumed. Just when Nancy's hair started growing back after radiation, she graduated to Adriamycin. Together, we grieved and worked through this second hair loss.

Throughout this difficult time we could watch the progress of her cancer by observing the ebb and flow of her skin cancer. Chemotherapy arrested its rapid spread but it did not push it back. When Adriamyacin appeared not to be helping, it was suggested she try a different chemotherapy, namely, Navelbine. Clearly each new drug was more toxic than the last.

The skin cancer was the overwhelming cause of Nancy's mental exhaustion. She had to face her cancer on a daily basis, look at it in the mirror, soak it in a urea solution for a half-hour, cream it down and then bandage it. She often said, "My brain tumor and liver tumors don't really bother me. I can't see them. Most days I can forget I have them. But my skin cancer is always right there, and it stinks!"

Daily she would ask me to look at it, help measure the field and comment on how it appeared to me. On top of her fatigue and nausea, this felt like one more thing which had wedged its way between us. Then too, I was now sensitive when I hugged her, careful not to squeeze her too hard, careful not to press the affected area too firmly.

One day, Nancy asked Margaux and me to sit down and talk. She knew it was time to die before the doctors did. She indicated she was totally drained and exhausted and she wanted to walk away from treatment. She didn't know how to tell us. She didn't want us to be angry with her. She didn't want us to be disappointed in her giving up the fight.

That day we talked, prayed and cried together, one loving supporting family. This conversation was extremely difficult for me as, at that point in time, I was the one struggling to let go. I did not want to let go of Nancy, even if it meant she was going to Heaven.

Within days of this pivotal discussion, Nancy took a sudden and dramatic turn for the worse. Yet another round of tests indicated the cancer had spread to the fluid in her spinal column. Now, the doctors said there was nothing more they could do for her. In her heart, she had the satisfaction of dismissing their treatments before they let her go. For me, it was a return to another crushing, repetitive cycle of hospital visits and another transfer to a nursing home.

Moreover, this time there was a major difference: the doctors said she had two months to live. Once again, they were wrong. This time she had just about two weeks.

She was fortunate at the end. She died at home. Peacefully. With very little pain, and very little medication.

The last few months of her life, I was under incredible pressure. I had lost my job and miraculously found a new one, thereby maintaining continuity in our health care benefits. I was torn between going to work and wanting to be with her. I was devastated, watching a person I dearly loved, die right in front of my eyes. Furthermore, I was frustrated by the limitations of support services and the frequent miscommunications that occurred in spite of everyone's best intentions.

From the moment a person is told they have cancer, the entire family is thrust on a roller-coaster of a journey. No one knows what lies ahead. No one knows how it will play out. There are countless decisions and revisions. Emotions run high, and low, in an endless, turbulent stream which can be likened to whitewater rafting.

This unique pioneering work, starting with the first diagnosis, provides intimate insights into a male caregiver's psyche, which in turn, helps women battling illnesses better understand what their loving male caregivers are experiencing. Then too, as stated earlier, stronger, more empathetic male support is priceless to any woman struggling with a major illness. The potential of this mutually beneficial synergy is endless.

Not everyone will want to read this book from cover to cover at one sitting. Rather, it is intended to accompany you through all the stages of your journey. Feel free to set it aside and to come back to it. Hopefully, you will be fortunate and after reading a few relevant chapters, you will be able to let this slender volume attract dust on your bookshelf. In that case, consider passing it along to someone else.

I hope and pray this book will support you and help you get through the inevitably difficult times. The longer and more intense Nancy's illness, the deeper our love grew. I loved her, cherished her, supported her and did everything I could for her. I wish you the same solace.

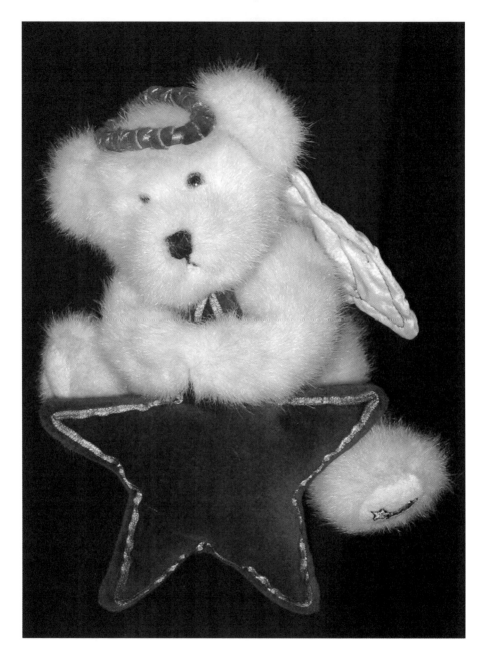

TABLE of CONTENTS

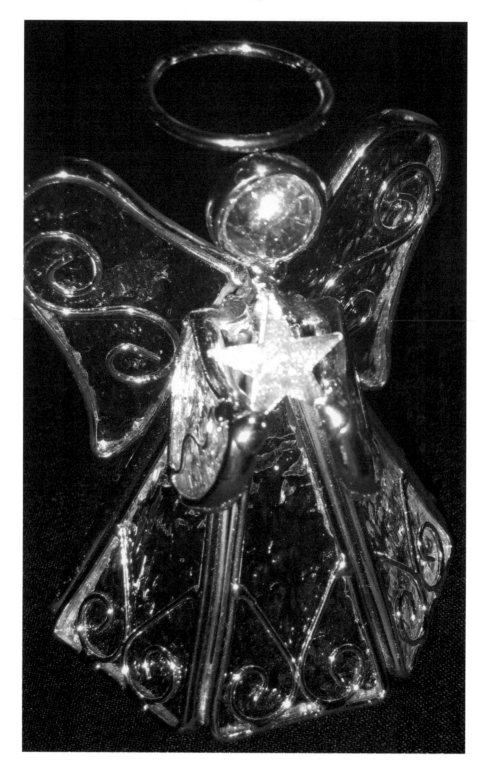

CHAPTER 1
The First Attack

"Breast cancer was a devious disease—a family of diseases, really, that began at the same site but behaved with frustrating variability. Or rather, with an incorrigible will: while patients talked about being survivors and marked each anniversary of their diagnosis, doctors always kept a wary eye on the horizon and spoke darkly of predestination. [Dr. Susan] Love had come to believe that there were three categories of disease: one third of all breast cancers were so virulent that they would kill a patient regardless of when the cancer was discovered or what treatment she had; one third were so indolent that they might laze around in the breast for years without posing a systemic threat; and one third existed in the middle ground—they required and responded to treatment. The only hope was to intrude on the process before the cancer colonized the liver or lungs or bone...metastatic cancer was incurable. Eventually it had its way."
To Dance With The Devil by Karen Stabiner.

The April sunrise was bright, clear and unexpectedly warm. After the deep dark snowy quiet of winter, the sound of chirping birds was strange and delightful to the ear. I rolled over and put my arm around Nancy. She snuggled back against the length of my body. I started massaging her neck and shoulders, expanding to long, sensuous caresses.

"Can I have a massage first?"

"Sure."

When I progressed to kissing her breasts, I noticed the left nipple was puckered and appeared inverted. I said something and she replied, "Let's worry about that later."

Little did we know our lives would never be the same from that moment on!

Nancy had a history of cystic-fibric changes, which meant she had lumpy breasts. She and I therefore took the inverted nipple seriously. The next step was a hurried appointment with our family doctor who had a pleasant low-key manner so we both felt at ease with him. After a brief discussion, he conducted a gentle but thorough examination and thought he felt a lump near the nipple. Nancy had brought along the x-ray films of the mammograms she had had done in New York City, shortly after we were married. While he encouraged us not to worry, he advised an updated mammogram and a biopsy in the very near future.

The discovery of a cancerous lump in Nancy's breast reminded me of an incident which occurred earlier in my life. I was a graduate student, living on New York's funky Lower East Side, when three youths came bounding up the tenement steps behind me. Intrusive. Threatening. When I turned to confront them, one put a knife to my throat and cautioned me to keep quiet. When I pushed him away, another beat me over the head with a cylinder. I fought back and made enough noise to cause them to flee. I walked away from the scene only to realize I was bleeding profusely. I spent three days in the hospital for observation. The scar on my chest and memories of the incident will remain with me the rest of my life. Like the thugs who assaulted me, threatening my life and taking something of value from me, when the hint of Nancy's cancer occurred, I not only felt instantly threatened and fearful again, but also deeply concerned for Nancy, our small child, Margaux, and for myself.

The biopsy was to be done at the hospital on an out-patient basis. Nancy had a choice between general anesthesia or a local anesthetic. She was positive she did not want to go under. She wanted a local as long as they assured her she would not be in pain. She was told she would hear what was going on and she would have some sensations, such as feeling pressure, but she would not have any pain.

4

I had an extremely uneasy feeling, the first of many. Then too, having to unexpectedly take time off from work for all these doctors' visits was intrusive. All of a sudden, life was not regular. I was worried about what would happen. Would I lose my wife at this young age? It seemed impossible to be left with a four-year old child, but such things did happen. This would be extremely difficult for me since I had no family in the area.

Then too, all of a sudden, our marriage and our close relationship had a different feel. Like the dark shadow of a solar eclipse, our sexual relations went on hold. Nancy was jumpy and irritable. It was difficult controlling my own emotions while supporting her at the same time.

Driving to the hospital for the biopsy, Nancy told me she did not want them putting her out under any circumstances. No matter what they said, she did not want any surgery other than the procedure we had discussed. I comforted her and told her not to worry. I assured her that no matter what happened, I was there for her. In my rush to help her, I soon realized I had made a promise which might be difficult to fulfill.

I stayed with her until they wheeled her near the entrance to the surgical area. The nurses then told me I would have to leave her and go to the waiting room. I gave Nancy a kiss and cheerfully told her I loved her and all would be well. However, deep down I felt both fear and panic.

After nervously pacing the waiting room for what seemed like an eternity, the attending doctor came out and informed me that the quick freeze test indicated the lump was malignant. I'll never forget the words, "It's cancer, but Nancy's doing well." Although given the option of waiting for definitive test results, the doctor recommended Nancy be administered general anesthesia for a modified mastectomy immediately, as she was already halfway under anesthesia. He said, "Doing it now will spare her going home, worrying about the surgery, and then going through all the pre-operative procedures again." Above all, he stressed that "it was imperative to act as soon as possible when it came to cancer." Although it sounded reasonable to me, I recalled our conversation in the car en route to the procedure. I felt as if I were living a bad dream, in real life. The worst case scenario was playing out. If I were in Nancy's position, I would seriously consider what Dr. Matins was recommending. However, Nancy's final instructions had been unequivocal. Therefore, I now had to find a way to keep this doctor from going further, even though it seemed logical to me. I felt tightly squeezed between two powerfully opposing forces.

I insisted we go and tell Nancy what was happening. While walking to the post-operative area I felt stressed and apprehensive. When questioned, Nancy had enough of her wits about her to tell Dr. Matins that she wanted to go home. He kept trying to talk her into a modified mastectomy but she said she wanted to go home. Period.

Back home, we sat in our living room in total shock. We hugged and cried together, then we talked. Nancy said she could feel the knife cut into her breast, yet, surprisingly, it did not hurt. She heard Dr. Matins say to a nurse, "This lump is hard. I'd bet anything it's cancer. Do the freeze test right away." It must have been so difficult for her to be treated as an object, for them to have discussed her condition as if she were not there.

He was so sure the lump was cancerous, Nancy questioned if they really did the quick freeze test procedure. She was appalled that Dr. Matins would push the surgery so aggressively. I then recalled our family physician had commented a quick freeze procedure could indicate cancer was present, when in fact it was not, or vice versa.

Nancy was adamant she never wanted to see Dr. Matins again. We decided to wait for the full test results and if it was necessary, she would pursue a second opinion with another surgeon. A short while later, the extensive test results confirmed the initial reading: malignant.

When first diagnosed, hearing the very word, "cancer", is like having a huge ice-cold dagger piercing your heart. Doctors tell you the condition can be treated and the survival statistics are impressive. Yet, a confrontation with the idea of death and mortality seems to over-ride any meager consolations.

An uncomfortably warm and humid weekend lay between Nancy's biopsy and her appointment with another surgeon for a second opinion. That Saturday afternoon, in shock, we sat on the patio while our daughter Margaux was taking a nap. I felt an inner turbulence yet, an uneasy sense of calm. Like a hummingbird hovering over a flower, pulsing its tiny wings at an incredible rate while appearing to be motionless, feelings, emotions and adrenaline were surging through our bodies. I remember lying out in the sun, numb with shock, seriously contemplating what life would be like for me without a wife, with no close family nearby and a dependent child. I was devastated. I asked Nancy how she felt.

She talked about second opinions for both the biopsy sample and the surgery. We discussed this at length, finally, talking about what was really on both our minds.

Nancy's mother had died when she was four years old. My father had died when I was four. The two of us shared the common experience of an unhappy childhood. At the age of four, there is almost nothing to hold onto after the painful finality of death.

I was distressed to face the reality, that in my heart, mind and soul, I had a blank where memories and images of my father would have been, had he lived. Except for their wedding picture, I had no idea what he looked like or what he enjoyed. Furthermore, I had no recollection of ever hearing his voice. Then too, my mother had always spoken of him in negative terms.

Margaux was four years old. We were riveted by the awful prospect of both our destinies' haunting the next generation. That Saturday afternoon Nancy and I bonded concerning an intense desire to spare Margaux a similar fate. We resolved to do everything we could. We did not know how we were going to do it, but we were going to fight cancer, if only long enough for Margaux to get to know her mother; long enough for her to have happy, loving memories. We had no way of knowing how long and how arduous the battle would become, yet, that fateful day we vowed to engage in it, together, to the bitter end.

We also talked about quality of life. We were determined not to let Nancy's cancer dominate our lives. Nancy wanted to be in control as much as possible and she wanted Margaux to have as normal a childhood as possible. The last thing Nancy wanted was for her to live in fear of the disease.

After the weekend pause, I had to return to work and we quickly returned to the task at hand. Our family doctor recommended a specialist in Philadelphia. The surgery would have to be performed in a center-city hospital. Nancy expressed concern for my having to drive such a distance. I told her to select her physician, then the hospital. Wherever it was, I would be there for her. Had I thought ahead, I would have realized it would be a logistical nightmare going into center city from the western outlying suburbs.

Furthermore, our four-year-old daughter required care but we had no family in the area. I gave little thought to this commitment too. I was simply doing what I felt should be done. Under such circumstances, it is easy to get into the habit of setting personal needs and requirements aside. This pattern was to continue and intensify over the years as we fought Nancy's illness. During the last two years of Nancy's life, it reached such acute proportions that I expressed virtually no personal preferences then, nor for years after her death.

The doctor's office was in a luxury high-rise tower. Extremely professional, he took time to review all the test reports and look at the x-rays. He discussed surgical procedures and answered Nancy's questions concerning possible breast reconstruction immediately following the amputation.

For my part, I found the concept bizarre. It seemed presumptuous for a mortal to claim the power to recreate a body part which had been removed. I thought the surgeon had an over-inflated ego. I asked about side-effects. We were shown photos of successful and unsuccessful reconstructions. The supposedly successful ones looked weird to me. All the photos of procedures gone wrong were frightening to me: skin that became necrotic, leaking implants. It seemed to me there were significant limitations and risks involved in such procedures and they were being minimized. I was uncomfortable with the possibility that Nancy and the surgeon would be keen over this operation when I personally would never consider it. However, if she wanted to do it, how vigorously should I argue against it? After all, it was her body and her life. Yet, the decision would leave an indelible imprint on me as well. In the end, she elected not to have reconstructive surgery done at the time of the mastectomy. I felt relieved.

Under pressure to act quickly, Nancy went with the second surgeon. Nancy was firm that she would not have done it any other way. Waiting for final test results and seeking the second opinion seemed prudent at the time. However, considering the precious time that had been lost, it worried me that possibly the cancer could be spreading and there could be detrimental side effects.

The surgery progressed predictably and relatively smoothly. My inner city skill of spotting parking spots was of great value.

After several days of recuperation in the hospital, I brought her home. It was about a forty minute drive and I remember avoiding potholes as if we were on eggshells. Although they had given her some pain-killers before we left the hospital, she could feel every bump in the road and every bump hurt. The next several days reminded me of when Margaux was born. Once again I was chief cook and bottle washer, taking care of both Nancy's needs and those of our daughter.

A day or two after she came home, we were together in our bedroom and Nancy asked me if I wanted to see her incision. The dressings had to be changed and this would be a good time. I said "sure" even though I felt very uneasy about it. If she was ready to show me, how could I say no? She slowly unbuttoned the large pajama top she had borrowed from me before going into the hospital. She positioned herself so I could see it and she could see me, yet she could also see the incision in the mirror. As she unbuttoned I asked her if she had seen it and she said she had not. She wanted me to look at it first. I asked her why she was peeking in the mirror and she said she wasn't peeking. She would look after I told her how it looked.

There was a long incision line over her left chest. Near her side there were still two holes where the post-surgical drains had been. I could see the stitches. I told her the stitches were black. She said the doctor told her they were black so they would be easy to find. It seemed to help her when I talked. Then she looked in the mirror and started crying. I held her close but very gingerly and I repeated that this did not detract in any way from her beauty as a person.

"How can you say that? I'm deformed. I look like a freak."

"Beauty is more than skin deep. This in no way affects how I feel about you. Margaux will not love you any less as a mother. Really, this is just not important. What is important is that you heal and get well and hopefully never have cancer again. If this is the worst that happens, we'll be lucky."

"It really doesn't bother you?" she asked. "You don't want to turn your head in disgust?"

"It really doesn't bother me. We'll make love and I'll prove it to you. Not today of course. I think it's best you heal and get the stitches out and then we can get really close."

In retrospect, I was delighted how natural and heartfelt my spontaneous responses were. However, looking back, it was indeed a greater issue for her than for me.

One incident, in particular, revealed Nancy's extreme discomfort concerning natural healthy breasts. Several years after her mastectomy, I purchased a plaster copy of the Venus de Milo. This headless, armless, legless torso of a woman had two wonderful breasts. Nancy virtually threw me and the statue out of the house.

We hugged gently and carefully. At the time, there was a sense of relief that this was behind us. Then she asked me if I would help wash her hair. The surgical area still hurt and she could not use her left hand. She suggested we could do it in the kitchen sink.

Margaux wanted to hug her mother, cling to her and squeeze her when Nancy first came home from the hospital. We therefore had to explain to Margaux, why she had to be so careful. When she asked "How long?" she was crestfallen to hear she would always have to be careful around her mother's left arm. Most importantly, however, Margaux had to be reassured over and over again that her mother would not die.

This extreme need to be careful around Nancy's left arm was also a major adjustment for me. For the first few weeks, I had to be careful rolling around in bed as Nancy was extremely protective and rightfully so.

About a week after the surgery we were called by our family physician. He regretted to inform us that test results indicated several lymph nodes were cancerous. This indicated the cancer had started to spread. The cancer had metastasized. He explained there was a possibility that cancer cells were circulating throughout her body. The only way to be sure of eliminating them, suppressing them, or driving them into remission, was chemotherapy. Nancy's initial reaction to chemo was negative. She denied the test results, asking about the degree of accuracy of the test. When informed the test was reliable, she questioned whether her tissue sample could have been mixed up with someone else's.

For me, this new development reaffirmed that the cancer was still a threat, even after Nancy's undergoing surgery. Furthermore, it was extremely challenging to contemplate still more time-draining doctor's appointments. I had already taken a lot of time off work with the tests, surgery and post-surgical care. Working for a leading department store, my boss had been very understanding and supportive. However, the work was piling up and I was falling behind on several important projects concerning government regulations and compliance. As I was involved in specialized, sensitive work, requiring attention to detail, there would be serious repercussions if something went awry concerning these work projects. However, Nancy was adamant that people at work should accept my absence during her weekly chemotherapy.

Nancy finally agreed to talk with an oncologist whose office was in center city in a row of old, tired buildings. This doctor was tall, slender and balding. Strangely cold, quiet and almost non-communicative, he seemed tired and burnt out. He spoke of his treatments as if they were the only thing to do.

Nancy asked him about radiation. He said radiation could accompany chemo but only chemo could get into the blood stream and touch all the cells with its protective qualities. He constantly kept referring to the lymph node involvement.

Eventually Nancy agreed to try low doses of chemotherapy. There was much discussion as to what constituted low dosage. She went for one treatment and spent the next week nervous and angry. She thought she could see her hair falling out after she combed it over the bathtub. She felt fatigued and in the waiting room she had heard talk about the cumulative debilitating effects of this particular treatment. We went back for the second appointment and her intense discussion with the doctor led to her decision to stop treatments.

I felt concerned, stressed and confused. It seemed to me that she was exaggerating the side-effects. It was as if she were looking for reasons to discontinue treatment. She discussed the situation with me at great length and I felt uncomfortable helping my loved one make a decision which could have life or death implications.

As she was going out the door, the chemo doctor insisted she should definitely have radiation but Nancy had stated clearly that she had had enough. Radiation was out of the question.

From the stress of the initial diagnosis through post-operative appointments, chronic fatigue had now became a part of both our lives. Unable to drive for about a month after her surgery, I continued in a supportive role, making time to drive her, and completing additional chores and errands she could not perform.

I tried to put myself in her position to understand how she felt. With my going off to work and Margaux in nursery school, Nancy faced long stretches of time coping with her illness, alone. Looking back, I really don't know how she did that. It seemed to me that loneliness could exacerbate the depression that follows the loss of a limb.

Nancy enjoyed visitors and accepted support from friends. She became active in local support groups such as Living Beyond Breast Cancer wherein she had positive interaction with others who were battling cancer. I actively sought to savor and enjoy every precious moment with Nancy and Margaux to the fullest.

After all we had been through, upon the advice of doctors and friends, Nancy made another appointment for us to see a local plastic surgeon with a fabulous reputation. We visited his office to further explore reconstructive surgery. The office was punctuated with large color photographs of patients before and after reconstructive surgery. There were noses, tummies, hips, lips and sundry other anatomical parts on display, including breasts.

The doctor sported an expensive suit and a full beard. He explained the techniques for reconstructive surgery.

Basically he inserted a synthetic implant or removed fatty tissue from another part of the body and implanted that under the skin. He could even take skin from another part of the body to fashion a nipple. We talked about the effect of reconstructive surgery on future mammograms and x-rays. It seemed to me that an implant could obscure efforts to detect possible future tumors.

He also talked about prophylactic surgery. This meant removing Nancy's other breast on the theory that it too might become cancerous. There were important statistics about how often additional tumors occur in the second breast.

To this doctor, prophylactic surgery meant a double reconstruction. If I found reconstruction bizarre, the thought of chopping off a perfectly healthy limb because another was diseased, almost sent me out of the room screaming. When Nancy and I had a chance to talk, I immediately made it clear I loved her with or without a breast. There was no way the absence of one organ could affect how I felt about her as a person.

As we leafed through a picture book, toward the end, the photos illustrated what could go wrong. The skin around an implant could die. Implants could leak. They could be rejected by the body. The doctor carefully described different implants and the specific reasons he selected the type he used.

Nancy decided not to have any further surgery at that time. I was relieved. Through a support group, Living Beyond Breast Cancer, she went to a local hospital and they helped her with a temporary prosthesis to place in her bra. It was a small hand-sewn bag filled with granules. She then made an appointment to be measured for a professional version. It was pink plastic filled with the material used in implants, molded to simulate her missing breast.

Rosalind MacPhee, a Canadian poet, in her book, *Picasso's Woman*, described the process of being fitted for and selecting a bra and prosthesis. When she found a swim suit that looked and felt right she stated, "A bathing suit told me symbolically that my life would continue to be active, as it had been before the surgery."

However, when a little camisole was suggested to my wife, Nancy, to help overcome initial shyness when first resuming love-making, she hurried out of the store. As expressed by Rosalind MacPhee, "My prosthesis lay on one side of the bed at night while my husband lay on the other."

The prosthesis was a major concern for Nancy along with major concerns about range of motion, regaining use of her affected arm in general, and the fear of a limb dangling useless. Swim suits represented another important subject. Nancy thought she would never look good in a swim suit again. Her surgeon assured her the scar would lie low and she would be able to wear even a low cut gown and a modest swimsuit.

In the midst of all these concerns, the loving partner is often left behind. Then too, sexual relations are often simply unattainable for psychological and physical reasons. However, supportive male care-givers need and deserve more consideration. MacPhee does not chronicle a discussion with her husband about how he felt about her appearance, about how he was impacted by her aches and pains. Nor did they discuss how he felt about less intimacy with her or what she might conceivably do to experience comfortable closeness and intimacy with him. Most men would welcome a conversation about what could be done for the woman without causing pain and discomfort. What might a woman enjoy after her painful traumatizing experience? What can her man do to bring a little joy, love and spice back into their relationship?

Now, here's what you can do.....

* Do not let anyone pressure you or your loved one into making quick decisions about additional procedures, tests, or examinations.
* Be careful not to make promises to your loved one that you can't necessarily keep.
* Obtain a second opinion in all major situations.
* Keep the lines of communication open with your loved one. Get in the habit of asking them how they feel about what is going on. In your own words, repeat what you heard them say, capturing the emotions as well as the content.
* Discuss your situation with your boss and co-workers. Stress at home can affect your performance on the job. Some individuals and co-workers will go out of their way to help. Others may be indifferent, taking the position, "I'm really sorry your spouse is ill; however, we have to get the work done around here." If in an unsupportive environment, be careful not to build up anger or resentment inside yourself.
* Recognize that stress leads to fatigue. Try not to become discouraged when fatigue becomes an integral part of your life.
* When going with your loved one to doctor's appointments, bring a note pad to take notes. Your spouse will often not retain a lot because they are in a mild form of shock. Typically, Nancy would ask me again and again what the doctor had said.
* If possible, avoid sitting too long in waiting rooms as negative conversations around you may often have very detrimental physiological effects on your loved one. My future friend, Lorna, would bring along special interest magazines, books and even personalized audio tapes to pre-occupy her ailing mother and father. It proved to be such a good side tracker that she later made personalized tapes for other friends who were battling chronic illnesses.

CHAPTER 2
The Aftermath, Fears, Tests

Charles was old enough to be my father and he more than looked the part with his bald head and broad Irish smile. Only a father would have taken on the responsibility of teaching a fellow from the streets of New York City, how to drive under snowy and icy conditions. Extremely skilled behind the wheel, he would often look into the rear view mirror and his whole body would twitch involuntarily. One time, driving on the New Jersey Turnpike, Charles talked about "rat-packing" and the danger of driving in the middle lane of a three lane, one way highway. Specifically, in the instance of a collision, cars in the middle lane had no place to go. Even the fast lane had only a half-shoulder. He felt the slow lane was safest because it provided the best option of a wide shoulder in the event of a problem. He then talked about a night in Chicago, "rat-packing", a chain collision, cars and wreckage all over the place. He recalled pulling an infant out of twisted metal. Tears came to his eyes as he relived the horror of death and blood all around, turning ordinary people into horrendous medical cases.

Cancer is just like that. Once told they have cancer, individuals will never be the same. It's as if they were destined to a lifetime of looking over their shoulder, looking in the rear-view mirror of life, fearing cancer may strike again at any moment.

After surgery and scores of follow-up appointments, although life was never quite the same as it had been before cancer intruded, sometimes it came quite close.

Gradually Nancy resumed driving and most of her interests. She proudly took Margaux to her first day at the elementary school and we lapsed into the rhythm of a regular, structured family life. Furthermore, at work, in addition to overseeing government regulations, I was put in charge of the central customer service area. This was a significant promotion, with a substantial increase in salary and the potential to advance to Vice President. Life was good again.

When Margaux became a little older, Nancy and I took a trip to Italy. It was one of those inexpensive, whirlwind tours with almost everything included. We went from Rome to Assisi, to Padua, to Venice, to Milan, to Florence and then finally, back to Rome. I fell in love with Florence and Rome. Right off, I declared that if I ever became rich and famous, I would move to Florence and buy a villa on the hill overlooking the Arno and the central tourist part of town.

Life was very good. We were doing so well we went back to Italy the very next year, taking Margaux along. This time it was an unescorted vacation. What a lucky eight year old to see such sights as the Sistine Chapel and soak in the beauty of Florence. In subsequent years we traveled to France, Spain, Germany, Austria and England. Most often we went as a family. Other times, Nancy and I would vacation ourselves.

Normalcy never returned to our personal lives but life went on. Nancy was involved in a whirlwind of activity. Looking back, I sense she used action and activities to dispel disquieting thoughts and feelings.

Like a sponge, I took it all in. Working at being a good listener, I refrained from sharing my innermost feelings. Thus, in addition to internalizing my frustrations and fears, I became even more considerate of her.

I sensed a high degree of anxiety each and every time doctors' visits approached. Although some individuals never suffer recurrence, follow-up examinations are a constant reminder that the threat is there. Just as the bottom of the ocean gets muddied by powerful passing storms, these exams, too, churn up feelings.

At such times, chances are, the person you are constantly supporting, may be irritable, moody, angry, preoccupied and even depressed. Like blinding rays of sun emerging from billows of dense dark clouds, the realization that cancer may be an incurable disease hits home once again.

A very close friend of mine once said, "My wife has a six-month follow-up exam after her diagnosis of cancer. I can't understand why she is so upset. It's just a routine exam." However, I quickly learned exams were never again to be routine. I was always intensely involved and extremely supportive around these doctors' visits.

As the battle against cancer is as much a psychological war of the mind as a physical and medical battle, it's of critical importance to keep spirits up and maintain a positive attitude. I found that confronting and accepting reminders that the disease can come back at any time, anywhere in the body, requires stamina, hard work and fortitude. The doctors will probably be positive and upbeat, but in the privacy of my innermost thoughts, there were many moments of fear, panic and anguish that things would never be the way they were, that someday my loved one might die a horrible death. On several occasions, I attempted to verbalize some of my feelings. Finding this not to be well received and somewhat hurtful to Nancy, I made a conscious decision not to discuss certain feelings with her, for fear of upsetting her or disturbing her equilibrium with her condition.

In general, Nancy and I managed, by and large, to keep our concerns between just the two of us. To the outside world it was virtually impossible to detect anything was going on.

Some men experience a feeling of helplessness when their loved one is faced with an incurable disease. Even more than feeling their hands are tied, some men feel completely bound, head to toe, frozen, trapped, and unable to move. Then too, most men are already not comfortable in the world of intense feelings, so they may experience helplessness while supporting their loved ones in this battle. Their entire world, like mine, can feel like it is spinning madly, wildly, totally out of control.

Another way your life may change will be around diet

and food. Nancy was always very interested in reading about her disease. She was keen about new research and recognized that recent literature made a compelling case for the role of diet in cancer prevention and fighting recurrence.

Consequently, Nancy started referring to foods in terms of their cancer-fighting qualities. Carrots were now "beta carotene." As she continued to investigate the subject, certain foods monopolized the family table. For example, I had always enjoyed broccoli, but, at one point, we were eating broccoli three times a day: broccoli omelets, steamed broccoli for lunch, and, the best for last, raw broccoli flowerets with dinner. Consequently, I lost my taste for broccoli. I could not eat it for years after Nancy's death. It took a long time to enjoy even an occasional mouthful. Then too during the last stage of Nancy's battle, she became nauseous around food smells in general. I later learned that my friend, Lorna, also experienced this food scent problem first hand when her mother was battling the final stages of breast cancer. However, as meals in general were still a highlight for her dad, she actually barbequed meals outside on a snowy patio so her dad could still enjoy his dinners without her mom having to suffer through the nauseous odors.

The more Nancy read about her disease, the more convinced she became that there was very little anyone really knew about cancer. No one could tell her what caused the disease. No one could guarantee a cure. No one could even reasonably assure her what to do to avoid recurrence. Being consciously, wholly supportive of Nancy's beliefs, I came to fully accept her point of view as the truth. Not until years after her death did my mind open enough to consider and accept other points of view.

Unfortunately, there's often a sense of shame or guilt attached to having cancer. People with cancer are embarrassed to have contracted the disease and feel that, perhaps, they did something wrong: improper diet, not enough exercise. Furthermore, if there is a history of cancer in the family, there may be a feeling of being the hapless victim. As the partner of a chronically ill person, I too, at times, felt guilty about being healthy. I wondered why I had been spared, when my loved one was suffering.

While Nancy continued her diligent studies, I was becoming more and more concerned about the financials. It's frightening to contemplate not having health insurance, yet millions of people are in that position. Since the odds of surviving cancer depend upon early detection, people without health insurance are at grave risk. Many chronic illnesses also debilitate the body, requiring extensive and expensive nursing and medical care. Unfortunately, some patients may not have health insurance that covers costly physical exams and test procedures.

The problem of out-of-pocket expenses was evident when I was at a breast cancer conference. During a break, I met a man searching desperately for a toilet. Attended mostly by women, the ladies had commandeered the rest rooms in general, pasting "WOMEN" paper signs over the men's rest rooms. Eventually we did find the one rest room the women had left for us. In the process we bonded over our wives' illnesses. This fellow had just started a business when his wife was unexpectedly diagnosed with breast cancer. When the dust settled, he had medical bills in excess of $75,000. He filed for bankruptcy, abandoned his business and commenced searching for a regular full-time job with health care benefits.

Little did I know, that in a few short years, I too, would be facing the prospect of losing my job and scrambling to find health care.

This issue was with me all the years Nancy fought cancer. It was my job to quickly learn the intricacies of our health care system and then, to work within it as much as possible. When a matter was of critical importance to her, I had to become adept at seeking exceptions to the rules. For example, Nancy might feel strongly that an MR exam required a repeat procedure as a second opinion. If the insurance company would not pay, I was often able to escalate her concerns to administration and secure approval of the second scan for her. Consequently, I spent countless hours obtaining referrals, questioning bills and calling the insurance company.

Another sensitive issue involves "significant others" being judged. For example, decades after my father died, I remember my mother recalling how the family blamed her for his death. Family members were adamant she could have done things differently. This judgmental atmosphere can, unfortunately, occur at any time during a serious illness.

Similarly, Nancy's mother died of breast cancer in her early thirties. Tragically, she left behind three small children. By the time she saw a doctor, the lump in her breast was so large the cancer had already begun its relentless spread. Thus, decades later, before and even after her husband passed on, family members wondered how he could not have noticed a huge lump in his wife's breast and openly vented their anger at him. He was still the scapegoat for their frustration, anger and unresolved feelings.

When your loved one has an incurable disease, you are already in a vulnerable, threatened position. The last thing you need is external second-guessing to stir up feelings of self-doubt and guilt.

While there are numerous support groups for individuals who contract serious chronic illnesses, are there effective groups for their supporters? Perhaps men are less likely to join support groups, as I observed very few men in the groups I attended. Consequently, there is clearly an ever growing need to encourage participation of men in support groups in general.

Short of men starting one for themselves, women can try to be more inclusive. For example, the grieving support group to which I belonged constantly distributed materials referring to "widows" but not widowers. When questioned, the response was: "One implies the other."

Happily, we've advanced well beyond the time when a speaker could address a gathering of men and women by saying, "gentlemen."

When a woman friend of mine volunteered to help at a major exhibit of breast cancer survivor art, her experience was that the women did little to invite, attract, or include men. In fact, they frequently, and inadvertently, said or did things which would discourage even those males who had been bold enough to express an interest in the subject.

Including "significant others" greatly benefits everyone. More than once Nancy phoned a cancer survivor only to be informed by the spouse that the woman had died. Nancy would then ask questions, and she became frustrated when the men did not share information. Perhaps if they had been included in support group activities, if there were more of a personal connection all along, there could be a willingness and ability for male caregivers to share more openly in general.

For example, once I was asked my opinion regarding a breast cancer support group fund raiser. The ladies had had several meetings and it seemed to me that most of the details had been finalized. There would be soft drinks, tea, sweets, a silent auction and a fashion show modeled by survivors. Finally, a female singer would perform. I took one look at the plan and expressed my amazement that men would be expected to attend. How many men would be comfortable and feel welcome with tea, diet coke and sweets on a Saturday night? Let the guys know they're wanted. Tell them there will be beer, wine and hors d'oeuvres. In any case, light alcoholic beverages could do wonders for bidding at the silent auction. My suggestion was implemented and the evening was quite the success. Then too, this group could have included a men's show in the fashion segment featuring a few of the supportive males.

Now, here's what you can do.....

* Most importantly, as the caregiver, utilize good listening skills to determine what your loved one needs, rather than progressing to actions which are based on what you think they need.
* Expect your actions to be judged by family and friends. Try and maintain your self-confidence and don't let anyone diminish it.
* Be patient and persistent when confronted with the maze of ever-changing insurance company rules. Never take "no" for an answer and do not be afraid to ask for an exception to the rule. From the very beginning, make it clear to the insurance company that you are discussing a serious situation and thus would appreciate higher level help.
* Establish a contact at a headquarter's level of your health care system and use that contact judiciously rather than for every little thing. Be polite, thankful and appreciative of any help received and make a point of praising health care employees for help received.
* If you feel you could gain strength from joining a group consisting of male care givers, ask your local hospitals for suggestions of where to find such groups, or possibly start one of your own.

CHAPTER 3
The Practical Consequences

Did you ever know a person who unfairly lost a job and then struggled to find a new job?

Cancer has the potential to toss you into a shadowy world of strange happenings; such as being denied insurance you desperately need, or being dismissed from a job for a reason which makes no sense at the time.

Power, money and politics. These eternal concerns impact individuals who are involved in a battle for their lives and the lives of their loved ones in unique ways. Some individuals become involved in the politics of the fight against cancer, striving to use their personal strength and power to direct the flow of government money towards finding a cure.

One October, when Margaux's godmother had come from Detroit to visit us, Nancy informed me that the two of them were joining the Pennsylvania delegation in the annual Breast Cancer March in Washington, DC. As I was not asked to go, I tentatively asked her if she wanted me to come along. She said it would be mostly women and that space was limited on the bus. Whereas part of me felt relieved about not going, a larger part of me felt disappointed.

Thanks to a series of photos Nancy took, I was later able to observe that thousands of women marched through the streets of our nation's capital. One huge pink and white banner proclaimed "Pennsylvania Breast Cancer Coalition- A Grassroots Effort." Individual placards stated "S.O.S. Save Our Sisters," and "Fund Breast Cancer Research." At one point there were huge puppet effigies graphically showing the scars and stitches following a mastectomy.

The foyer to the White House was a surrealistic scene. It reminded me of a Jean Luc Goddard movie, where an incredible traffic jam brought thousands of cars to a halt, resulting in a seething tumultuous panorama of life. It looked like a major political party's nominating convention.

There were placards with the names of individual states and the number of signatures collected in each: "Utah, 10,600," "Virginia, 62,400," and "Maryland, 48,200." A huge tractor trailer was draped with a massive banner, "END THE BREAST CANCER EPIDEMIC." Under the ribbon were hundreds of file boxes, labeled by state, containing millions of signatures of women who had been touched and maimed by this horrible disease.

Nancy came home exhausted, yet flushed with a sense of accomplishment. She had successfully played her part in creating the tapestry of a historic moment which was to echo and reverberate for years to come. Later, I learned that The National Breast Cancer Coalition (NBCC) had been trying to get into the White House to present their case for years. They made it on October 18, 1993 and Nancy was there with them.

Had I been invited and thus been a part of this, could I have possibly gained some much needed strength and energy to help me support Nancy even more? Could I have been exhilarated in the moment by the bonding group achievement rather than learning about it secondhand? Did I have to comprehend the visual impact days after the fact through photographs? After all, I had most sincerely offered to be involved.

This glimpse into the political aspect of the fight against disease contains an important lesson for men with afflicted loved ones. Debilitating, incurable diseases, initially touch one person and then the effects reach out and seriously scar many more. Thus the presence of male caregivers can strengthen marches such as these in many ways. As men, we need to be involved: for our loved ones, for ourselves, for our relatives, friends, neighbors and, above all, for our children.

Engaged in a fight with a life-threatening illness,

bodies and minds are stretched to the limit, both at home and in the workplace. Gradually, more and more often over the dinner table, Nancy started discussing frustrating difficulties with her present boss. Eventually, she was asked to leave this position.

A boss can be intimidated by the prospect of recurrence, time off for surgery or treatments, and large chunks of sick days, all of which disrupt the flow of an already stressed work environment. Then too, in private, Nancy questioned possible intrusions into her private data: "Just how confidential are my medical records when they run background checks? And, if it's a move from one position to another within the company, who's to keep the hiring manager from looking through my medical file?"

The confidentiality of health records is indeed a major issue and a subject all in itself. When I worked in Delaware, one of my associates, a Vice President with a long, successful record with the company, counseled me during an open enrollment period. "You know I've had open heart surgery. I will never be able to buy life insurance. It's not right. Statistics show many people live long full lives after heart surgery, especially when combined with exercise and diet. I feel better now than I did for years before the surgery. Take a good look at this new insurance benefit. Buy all you can for your wife. It's probably the only chance you'll have. Sure, there's such a thing as an assigned risk pool, but the premiums are astronomical. It's not practical. Me, I'm signing up for the maximum. No medical exam, no restriction for pre-existing conditions. You have to do it."

Now, here's what you can do.....

* Try to re-structure your finances as if you were the sole wage earner. This will reduce your stress should you find yourself in that position.
* Study the fine details of your health care plan. Be polite but assertive in seeking exceptions when they are required.
* Understand that your ability to change jobs or pursue your career can be substantially impacted in subtle and complex ways. For example, if a rival firm offers you a lucrative job on the other side of the U.S., you must determine whether your health coverage applies in that geographical area. Many HMOs are regional. A new HMO in another region might require a one-year waiting period for pre-existing conditions. If you make that career move and your spouse has recurrence, you might very well be looking bankruptcy in the face. Furthermore, changing health plans under such circumstances can be a risky proposition. Should you have to change plans, seek reassurance about pre-existing conditions and get it in writing.

CHAPTER 4
Recurrence

"Can we touch it?" The scent of formaldehyde was in the air. The small blue lump was in a plastic tray in front of us. Nancy and I were in the basement of our local hospital, in the Pathology Department, asking to examine the tumor that had been removed from her breast during her mastectomy nine years earlier.

Several times in my life I have experienced situations where I had the eerie feeling I had previously lived or experienced a particular moment. Facing recurrence is just like that, except the situation is a horrible nightmare, accompanied by heart-pounding, gut-wrenching fear, anger and anxiety.

About seven years after Nancy's first surgery, during one of her follow-up appointments, the doctor felt a lump along the surgical line. As she had already passed the five year mark and statistics indicated that most people who pass this milestone without recurrence have excellent prospects of living a life free of cancer, this was a real shocker. Our normal rhythm of everyday life was suddenly disrupted again. We scrambled to get a second opinion and to find a surgeon we trusted.

The surgery went without incident, except for one inescapable fact: the cancer was back! This time it was very challenging for me in a different way as our daughter, Margaux, now was old enough to understand the gravity of the situation. Consequently, not only did I need to support Nancy through her surgery but I also needed to guide our ten year old daughter through all her fears and uncertainties.

Accordingly, on the day of the surgery, I had to summon the strength to both part with Nancy at the door of the surgical unit and assure Margaux that her mom would not die in surgery, that her mom would come back home.

Now, all three of us had to process this new reality. We went from the prospect of a life without cancer to the frightening realization that there were more cancer cells in Nancy's body. No one could tell when they would act up and attack us again. Hopefully the lump had been successfully removed. However, once again her entire body was at risk and our world was turned upside down.

In addition to this most recent discouraging medical development, Nancy was angry with me. I had been out of work for more than a year as I had lost my Divisional Vice President job due to a corporate reorganization. It was the worst time of my life. I was extremely stressed out. When I did go back to work, I had half the responsibility and half the pay we used to enjoy so Nancy, too, had to go back to work. She claimed she was doing all the right things: close monitoring, proper diet and exercise. Thus, she blamed me for the recurrence. She believed that my problems intruded on her life, and, furthermore, she felt that the resultant stress I heaped on her probably caused her cancer to return.

On top of all this, Margaux was now about ten years old, whereas at the time of Nancy's first surgery, Margaux was only four. Consequently, this time, during numerous family discussions concerning her mother's cancer, she was frightened and needed immediate and constant consolation. She was afraid her mother would die. Margaux was told that it was just a recurrence along the old surgical line, and that we were fortunate her mother had opted for six month follow-ups. Happily, the cancer had been caught early and prospects were excellent it would all be removed. However, Margaux wanted to know why the cancer had come back. She wanted to know if it came back once, could it come back again?

I quickly learned there was a fine line regarding what to say to a child and what not to discuss. This line varies based upon age, maturity and other circumstances. When discussing serious illness with children, care must be taken to consider both the present and the future.

What happens, what's discussed and the manner in which situations are handled, will have long range implications.

The direct blunt child questions rang Nancy's bell. Sensing that all of Nancy's concerns and fears were touched by Margaux's simple pointed questions, I tried to help answer them factually, yet to temper the response in such a way as not to cause undue concern or fears. We also met with the guidance counselor at school and clued him in on what was occurring. He went out of his way to meet with Margaux and discuss what was on her mind.

Somehow, I had to find the inner strength to both support Nancy and help Margaux cope with her fears and concerns, all the while juggling the extensive demands of my job. Margaux had support at school and Nancy was very active in local breast cancer support groups; however, I was going it alone. There was no family in the area for much needed external support and not only was I feeling the sting of Nancy's anger, I was beginning to feel more and more guilty in general.

Nancy went back to her pattern of twice-a-year examinations, sometimes even more frequently than that. The slightest suspicion of anything out of the ordinary would send her back to the doctor's office. Furthermore, as the second surgery thickened her surgical line and added more scar tissue to her left chest area, self-examination for lumps was extremely problematical.

Often she would ask me to feel an area she thought was suspicious. I felt extremely uncomfortable being asked to do this. Already she was blaming me for her recurrence. What if I should fail to detect a lump or thickening? As I was not trained and did not know precisely what to look for, I was in the uncomfortable position of wanting to help, yet realizing I was inadequate for this responsibility.

During a follow-up appointment with her surgeon, Nancy asked if it would be possible to see any of her

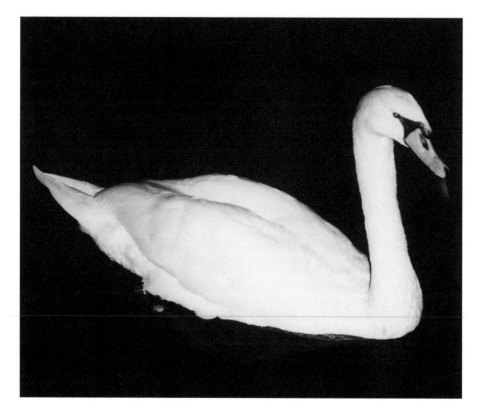

To appreciate the ying and yang of my situation, envision a stately swan, gliding seemingly effortlessly, along a tranquil lake. However, just out of sight, beneath this calm tableau, the webbed feet of the swan are paddling furiously.

tumors. Her physician responded without hesitation that this could be easily arranged. Accordingly, that afternoon we went to the pathology department of the local hospital. Not surprisingly, it was in the basement. I fought back scary images of a morgue-like setting where dead bodies were brought to await the local under-taker.

However, this pathology department was brightly lit and incredibly bustling. At the reception desk, we were asked to wait a few minutes while the specimen was pulled from the archives and prepared for our examination.

Shortly afterwards we were ushered into a small room and directed towards a glass jar, labeled with Nancy's name, date of surgery and data on the type of tumor. The technician used tweezers to pull a small lump out of the jar and she placed in on a plastic tray.

"Why is it blue?" Nancy asked.

"Specimens are dyed to facilitate examination under the microscope. We also have slides of your tumor. Would you like to see them?"

"Sure." Turning to me Nancy said, "Anthony, do you want to touch it? It's okay if you don't want to..."

"Sure, I'll touch it." I was amazed at how hard and dense the tissue felt. Immediately I could understand what all the doctors were feeling for when they did manual examinations. Dense and hard, you could almost call them angry tight balls of flesh.

It was as though Nancy had finally come to face her nemesis after all these years, *mano y mano.* She could see it, touch it, talk to it. It was a positive, liberating experience for her. Me, I would not have gone to the basement, let alone touch the specimen. However, I did it, because she needed to do it, and I wanted to be there for her, to provide support.

Personally, I found it very awkward but I could not help but think, 'What an incredibly brave woman! How creative to want to confront your illness and mortality in this manner and stare right at it. I don't think I would have ever thought of doing it.'

Shortly after this, Nancy grudgingly returned to full time work. From then on, whenever the three of us gathered at the dinner table, she would often talk about how difficult her days were and how much full-time work took out of her, when she most needed all her energy to fight her cancer. I felt guilty about Nancy's stating her fear that pressures on the job could cause yet another recurrence and I offered to work two or three jobs so she could stay home and heal herself. She refused on the grounds I would be miserable and complain all the time. Not only did I feel bad I was earning only a fraction of what I had previously earned, but, in addition, I felt frustrated and helpless because this was having such an overwhelming impact on my family.

Sure enough, less than two years after her second surgery, the doctors found another nodule along the surgical line. This time it was even more serious. The cancer had penetrated deeper and the tumor was partially attached to the muscle of her chest wall. Although it would be outpatient surgery again, this time the recovery would be more painful and drawn out.

This news precipitated another round of recriminations. Nancy was even angrier after this most recent recurrence. I felt guiltier and fought back intense feelings of frustration. Margaux was more frightened than ever her mother was going to die. Now a teenager, she was experiencing the pain of how cancer could spread. Its awesome power had become clear.

After these three surgeries, they then discovered yet another tumor in Nancy's chest wall. Nestled under the clavicle bone, this tumor was inoperable. The good news was that radiation and chemotherapy could eradicate it. Nancy opted for the radiation but once again refused chemo.

After three weeks of radiation treatments, the already damaged skin on her left chest had now become red, an indication of still more damage. At that time, there was no way for us to know how crucial a role this skin damage would play in the future.

Then, there was still more recurrence, spreading to the bones of the spine. Now I heard the phrase for the first time: "breast cancer sometimes goes to the bones." All the cancer specialists were aware of this. However, until it actually happened, no one discussed it with us. I understood the gravity of our situation when I was told the cancer could so weaken the bone structure that patients often fractured their spines simply getting up out of a chair.

This necessitated another round of radiation. Once again Nancy refused the recommended chemotherapy. This time the skin on the small of her back just above the buttocks turned permanently red.

Through it all, we went out of our way to enjoy life. We tried to keep up our annual European vacation and I included Nancy and Margaux in my business trips whenever possible. As a result, I can look back at our happy times in such wonderful cities as San Francisco, Chicago, Washington DC and Nashville.

I recall just one trip when Nancy was too ill to travel. It was January and I had to go to Houston. As Nancy had just started radiation therapy, she was not only too weak to go with me, but, also, could not miss any treatments. We therefore made arrangements for her to stay with our very dear friends, Julie and Jack, with whom Nancy felt very comfortable, and I left for Houston in a snowstorm and returned just ahead of another. In fact, the moment I landed, it started snowing.

I jumped in my car and made it safely home, but that night on the news, I learned that climactic conditions had spawned extremely icy conditions in the area around the airport. Numerous accidents had occurred literally minutes after I passed through.

God took care of me as Nancy needed me back home safe and sound that night. I had important work to do.

Now here's what you can do.....

* Recurrence represents a crucial milestone for everyone involved. The loving partner should try to reduce stress by any means possible.
* Try not to let recurrence wedge itself between you and your loved one. Work at becoming closer, taking full advantage of every opportunity to live life to the fullest.
* Maintain open lines of communication. Include children in discussions, so that everyone knows each other's fears and concerns.

CHAPTER 5
Intense Stages

Once, at the Jersey shore, I was wading in water up to my chest when a wave knocked me over and the current pulled my feet out from under me. My whole world was topsy-turvy. I reached for the bottom and felt water. My head bumped against sand where there should have been air and sky. In a panic, I started swallowing salt water when I should have been sucking in good clean air. For a brief moment, I thought I was going to die. In the end I lost my glasses and my swim trunks.

So it is when cancer starts to roll though the body of a person you love, except that the fear, anguish and disorientation are extremely protracted. There is precious little time to regain your equilibrium and your strength when you are tossed head over heels again and again. The net effect is exhausting and debilitating.

The signs were barely noticeable at first. Like one neon sign on the Las Vegas strip, the first warnings were lost in the hustle and bustle of what we call 'the Holidays.' Around Thanksgiving, Margaux came home from college to visit and, together, we noticed Nancy was becoming forgetful. Specifically, she would start a sentence and forget the ending before she could say it:

"Anthony, will you go to the food store and get some..."

"Get some what?" I would ask her after a respectful pause.

"Get some...(another pause) I can't remember!"

At first we attributed it to encroaching middle age, perhaps even general forgetfulness. It did not seem to get any worse, yet, it wasn't getting any better after the New Year.

That December, for example, when Margaux had come home for the holidays, she too noticed her mom's forgetfulness had worsened. One day, when they had gone to the mall, it was as if her mother were in another world. "I would be talking to her and she would be really out of it," Margaux recalls. "She was spacey, she was not talking at all. She seemed to be a different person, quiet, not her usual self." At that time, Margaux and I discussed Nancy's memory loss at length and concluded it was significant, but we were at a total loss to understand what it meant.

After the holidays, Nancy was intent on seeing a specialist in New Jersey regarding the edema in her left arm. Before this, without fail, I would have driven her. However, that morning, there was a particularly important reorganization meeting at my bank. Word was out that there were thousands of positions slated for elimination. Consequently, at the last moment, Nancy called several individuals in her support group and as no one was available to drive her, she went on her own.

That afternoon the phone rang and Nancy was in tears. Angry and frustrated, after arriving and discovering the doctor was not in that day, she had bumped into a parking divider and seriously damaged her car. She was frightened, as she did not remember turning the car on. Nor did she remember hitting anything. However, all of a sudden, she had become aware of major damage to the front fender and hood.

Initially, I was understanding and supportive, asking if she was okay. When I heard she was not hurt, I reassured her that cars can be fixed. Deep down however, darn it, I could not help but be upset because she was driving our brand new car. Thus, although I was primarily concerned about Nancy, I was also upset, yet not able to be upset, about the car. I was also suffering through a major upheaval at work. Now I felt guilty again; if only I had driven her, none of this would have happened.

The issue of driving is extremely sensitive for all parties. In Pennsylvania, it is a law, that individuals undergoing radiation treatments to the head, are not allowed to operate a motor vehicle. The legal and insurance ramifications of a person with a brain tumor getting in an accident are awesome. Consequently, the driving falls upon the care provider. Frequent doctors' visits and treatments, make it all the harder for the caretaker to keep up with work commitments. Friends, church and support groups can therefore be an invaluable resource during such difficult times. Nancy, however, by choice depended mainly on me.

Then, in January, Nancy talked about pain in her lower back. First she had an MRI and the results were negative. Her specialist ordered a CAT scan of the liver, just as a precaution, just to be sure. Unbelievably, the CAT scan indicated multiple tumors of the liver.

While meeting with an oncologist, I mentioned the forgetfulness. I asked if anything further should be done. We were told not to concern ourselves; chemotherapy would take care of the liver tumors and any other tumors that might exist. Although I was extremely uncomfortable with this situation, I did not want to challenge her doctor or push the issue and upset Nancy more.

A day or two later, our family doctor called to discuss the scans and the liver tumors. After talking briefly about the liver, I then pressed forward, once again, with the issue of forgetfulness. I asked if she should have a scan of the head to rule out any problems. Our family doctor said he would speak with the oncologist.

The next day, my anxiety had increased to intolerable levels. I took it upon myself to call Nancy's radiation oncologist. As soon as I explained the situation, she was quick to concur that a CAT scan of the head was definitely in order. As it turned out, Nancy had a brain tumor which now represented a more immediate and serious threat to her than the liver tumors.

I was glad and relieved I had pushed to find out what was really going on. I was also devastated. The speed with which the cancer struck at two vital organs was overwhelming. In a flash the fact that she was dying and

I might lose my job became all too real. How was I going to tell Margaux? How was I going to handle all this by myself?

The first radiation treatments to the head showed no outward results. However, after a week or two, her hair started to fall out and Nancy complained about excessive hair loss when she brushed her hair each morning. As her hair was her crowning glory, her one major indulgence had been, through good and bad times, a weekly appointment at the hairdresser's. Thus it was extremely upsetting for her when her hair started falling out in clumps.

I, too, soon noticed long strands of hair all over the house. Each morning our bed seemed full of hair. To help her cope with this loss, Nancy asked me to gather up handfuls of hair, go out on the front lawn and cast them to the wind saying, "Come back to Nancy when her radiation is finished." This little ritual helped her, but it was of little comfort to me.

From a practical standpoint, there was no one for me to talk to about this most recent development. I could not tell Nancy how upsetting the whole thing was for me because it would just make her feel bad. I could not discuss the matter with Margaux as she was away at school and Nancy did not want her to know. Nancy would explain it to her when she came home to visit. Furthermore, I was warned not to discuss such details with Margaux under any circumstances.

Nancy started wearing a turban. At one point she asked a friend of the family, a registered nurse, to come over and shave her head because she could not stand it any more. Our friend arrived with scissors and razors. She and Nancy chatted for a long while before Nancy took off her turban and Linda took a look. Linda was adamant that shaving Nancy's head, as they do prior to surgery, was the wrong thing to do.

Over the next few days Nancy became increasingly uncomfortable and irritable over her hair loss. I suggested she make an appointment with her stylist, to at least have it washed, but Nancy complained it was not worth the money as it was falling out too quickly. Finally, I talked her into it, and it was one of the most important things I ever did.

Nancy's stylist, Diane, was very relaxed and calm. She offered to wash Nancy's hair herself rather than leave it to an assistant. As Diane washed, she massaged Nancy's scalp. Nancy said it felt very good. Immediately, Diane and I could see that rooted hairs and hair which had fallen out were all intertwined. Then it appeared as if the whole top of Nancy's head was coming off.

Patiently, Diane kept working the mass until she had removed just about all of Nancy's hair in one big wad. She silently questioned me what to do with it. I motioned her back to discard it, obviously without Nancy's seeing it. At the end, Nancy sat in the chair and Diane trimmed the few hairs left on the nape of her neck. Nancy looked at herself in the mirror and cried. Then she stopped crying because, I think, she did not want to upset Diane. I gave Diane a whopper of a tip.

Several months later I asked Diane how she felt performing that service for Nancy. She said it was no problem. I suggested she might be able to help other cancer patients in this manner.

On the way home I treated Nancy to a ride back through horse country. We seldom drove that way and she enjoyed it even though she was exhausted. It was great to give her some relief and comfort. In the moment, I didn't even notice that there was little or no relief for me. I didn't have time to observe that I was depleting my energy reserves at an incredible rate.

Between the radiation and the decadron to reduce swelling of the brain tumor, Nancy became progressively weaker. She started to take long rests and naps between activities. Then, even her legs started to buckle under her.

At the outset we were told that radiation therapy treatments could not be missed or postponed. It was winter. She asked me to drive her to each and every treatment.   Fortunately, my boss at work was understanding and sympathetic. However, this did little to allay my fears, should severe snow or ice storms occur.

During the last few days of her three weeks of treatment, a major snow storm was predicted for the very last day. When I awoke that morning, storm warnings were in effect and a light snow had started to fall.   I couldn't help but recollect a serious car accident I had been involved in, twenty years before this snowy scenario.   As I was critically injured and thus was hospitalized for twenty-one days, I have tried, ever since that time, to avoid driving in icy and snowy conditions, unless absolutely necessary.

Therefore, the morning in question I felt extremely troubled as I was not only struggling with my own memories, but I was also genuinely concerned for Nancy's welfare on any slippery surfaces. However, when I called the radiation center, they said they were open and would take her as soon as we got there.

By this time she had become so weak it took a long time to help her get dressed.   I was extremely apprehensive as we walked onto our snow covered patio and approached the car. Her legs were so undependable that she would have to aim her bottom at the car seat and collapse. She insisted I bring her handbag and she showed me a copper bracelet Margaux had received from her boyfriend.   Margaux had gone back to college and Nancy had talked them into having it engraved. Nancy insisted on taking care of it that very day because Margaux was so busy at school.

I drove carefully through the snow and we arrived at the radiation center without incident.   When her treatment was completed, Nancy received a certificate of completion. She was exhausted, but happy and relieved to be finished.

No sooner did I get her out of the wheelchair and into the car, when she demanded I drive her to the local trophy shop to have the bracelet engraved. It was not far from the house, but the snow was coming down harder and harder. I therefore firmly told her I would take her home and I would then drive to the store alone. However, she insisted that I take her with me. She would not take no for an answer.

The roads were now snow covered and slippery. When we arrived at the trophy shop, we were confronted with several extremely treacherously slippery wooden steps. Although I almost had to carry her, she still insisted on going in. As it turned out, the trophy shop did not do engraving of this sort and suggested we take the bracelet to a jeweler. When Nancy asked which one they recommended, the lady mentioned a shop which was all the way back in the direction of the radiation center.

I insisted on taking Nancy home. I told her to forget about the bracelet on such a stormy morning. Again she refused. She berated me angrily to take her there or she would drive herself, no matter what. After the jewelers, we went home and, still angry, she collapsed. She was furious I had given her such a hard time over such an important matter.

Upset and confused, Nancy really did not mean what she said, yet, it hurt, and there was nothing I could do other than just deal with it. In order to make it through this stage, I learned to frequently leave the room for awhile, taking time to recompose myself. This eerie scenario would recur time and time again.

I missed a lot of time at work. It felt as if I were stuck in quicksand and couldn't get out. Each morning we would get up and assess the situation. Bottom line, she needed me and could not be left alone.

One day I felt a nasty virus coming on. I knew I just couldn't get sick. By sundown I was running a temperature of one hundred and three. I got Nancy into bed, staying as far away from her as I could. I then focused on the bad germs and tried, through concentration, will power and sheer determination, to drive them out of my body. I remember getting very hot during the night and sweating profusely. When I awoke the next morning I felt weak, drained and empty, but I had no fever and I carried on as if nothing had happened.

Valentine's Day occurred during this difficult and challenging time. I was not sure Nancy would have the strength to celebrate. However, even in the midst of grave adversity, we always found a way to have fun and enjoy life. This Valentine's Day was one of those unforgettable experiences.

After a brief discussion, it was clear Nancy wanted to go to our favorite Italian restaurant in Malvern, "Anthony's". As this establishment did not take reservations and she was too weak to wait for a table, I called and asked to speak with the owner, Anthony. I explained our circumstances. He reiterated the policy of not reserving tables. However, he kindly assured me that if we got there around five o'clock, before six p.m., a table would be held for us.

We started getting ready early. Nancy's weakness had intensified and I totally misjudged the amount of time it would take me to dress her. I had to put her socks and shoes on, and help her pull up her pants. It was a struggle but we made it to the restaurant while our table was still available.

Nancy was so happy to be there. Joy beamed and radiated from her face. We talked while we waited for our food and I had them open the wine and light the candle on the table. "La bella luna," she said, "La bella luna." This was a line from Moonstruck, one of our favorite movies. We had seen it again and again. I turned around and looked out of the frosty sweating windows and sure enough, there was the full moon. It was as if the silvery rays were magically transforming Nancy's tired worn face into one of joy and satisfaction. For a while, that night, we were both happy and at peace.

Life was an emotional roller coaster. The very next evening Nancy took offence over some perceived slight and became extremely angry with me. She had unintentionally crossed over the line to verbal abuse. She was screaming and yelling, ranting and raving. At wit's end, I called her radiation oncologist. When the answering service came on I was emphatic it was indeed an emergency. By the time the doctor called back, the situation was totally out of control. The doctor tried one tack, then another. Finally she told Nancy, "Stop worrying about different things. Get in bed and make love with your husband." Nancy found this humorous and laughed. Her laughter had a strange tone to it and the entire incident was hauntingly unnerving for me. Nancy was to tell the story of this phone call over and over again.

Another gut wrenching day of my life occurred when our cousins visited for a weekend. They had left Sunday night to drive back home and that Monday morning, Nancy awakened, determined to unwrap all the good china and crystal. I could not understand why. Something felt dreadfully wrong. We had been going through a phase during which she would have intense anger, and berate me, bully me, intimidate me and threaten me.

I was freezing up. As I froze up, her anger intensified. She screamed at me to do this and that. Reluctantly I pulled down boxes of our precious crystal, hands shaking, while she ranted at me.

Finally, I blew the whistle. I told her something was going to bust: me, the crystal, or both.

After a lot of emotional upheaval she finally said, "I am going to serve my cousins on MY good china and crystal and silver, no matter what happens."

I said, "I told you your cousins went home last night."

"What day is this?"

"It's Monday."

"I thought it was Sunday."

Her memory loss had struck again. Then we went into the unpleasant reoccurring scenario during which she felt the fear and guilt of screwing up what day of the week it was, and me, I had all the hurt and pain. Not only was I trying to cleanse myself of her anger and venom, I was frightened over what was happening to her mind. I felt so alone, with all my fears, which I knew I could not discuss with her.

Several days later, in the morning, Nancy could not get out of bed. She could not move at all. She said she was ready to be admitted to the hospital. After making a round of calls to the family doctor and the radiation oncologist, hospitalization was quickly arranged.

I offered to call the local volunteer ambulance company for assistance, but Nancy was adamant that I would drive her. Although we had contributed to the local ambulance group for years and had never used the service, Nancy would hear nothing of it. I was concerned about both her getting in and out of the car and my ability to support her with my sore back. It took her a long time to get ready and before we left she insisted on her usual breakfast of two eggs over lightly with coffee and toast.

When I got her to the emergency room at the local hospital, the admitting doctor had left orders for a series of tests and I remember the technician not being able to find a vein. Hours went by as one IV unit after another gave it a try. Finally they asked me to leave and I believe a doctor or surgeon drew blood by cutting into an artery in her groin. It was explained that Nancy could not be admitted without the blood tests.

Her first day in the hospital was grueling and draining. I must have looked like I was going to collapse as the nurses kept telling me to go home. I was anxious to take their advice when it was announced that the chief oncologist would be making the rounds. If I could wait a little while longer, he would take time to talk with me. Whereas, my best interests would have been served if I had gone to bed, I felt Nancy needed me to meet with the doctor. Therefore, I waited it out.

This doctor wore very expensive custom-made suits. He took me to a small, private meeting room where we had a chance to talk. When he asked me what Nancy's wishes were should her heart stop or should she stop breathing at night, I did not know what to say. We had never talked about this. I then realized she was worse off than I had suspected.

However, after a few days in the hospital, the rules required she be discharged. This was my first confrontation with a medical system that did not seem to want to hear that I could not take care of her by myself. I felt threatened and bullied when they talked about discharging her at a specific day and hour. Eventually, someone clued me in to the fact that she could go to a nursing home. Thus, in a matter of hours, I had to research a few local nursing homes and make, on her behalf, extremely major personal decisions.

Most people take weeks, if not months, to make such important decisions.

Entering a nursing home for the first time, with a middle-aged spouse, who is incapacitated on a stretcher, and debilitated by cancer treatments, is like suddenly finding yourself in a foreign land, where the people, food, language and currency, are completely strange and unintelligible. I personally encountered many elderly individuals confined to wheelchairs, some babbling incoherently, others hallucinating over perceived wrongs. Should you find yourself in such a position, do yourself a favor and ask a friend to go with you.

You will soon discover nursing homes are a regulated industry and you will be subjected to a mountain of complex forms. At best, it takes over an hour for the nursing home administrator to explain the forms to you and then insist that you sign each one.

There are serious financial consequences to many of these forms. Other forms can dramatically impact the type of care your loved one receives, should an emergency arise. I felt completely overwhelmed, suddenly placed in the difficult position of making numerous quick decisions which would affect Nancy's life and our present and future financial well-being.

The subject of a living will is also inevitable. Under any circumstances, this is a very complex subject with grave potential outcomes. You should not allow yourself to be coerced into hasty decisions, as in all likelihood, these matters will unfortunately demand your attention when you are pitifully short of time and energy.

In our case, a nearby nursing home, in a highly regarded community, seemed reassuring at first. Psychologically, I needed a respite of sorts. I needed and hoped for a small degree of relief from the role of sole care-provider, a break from weeks and months of unending stress.

However, my needs were not to be met. Rather than having pleasant and somewhat relaxed visits with Nancy each day, I, instead, was confronted with nonstop complaints. Amongst other things, Nancy said the nurses were making fun of her slurred speech. She was humiliated, having to ask strangers to help her get on the bedpan.

Furthermore, she felt people in general spoke disrespectfully to her and voiced that the nurses were slow to respond to her flashing signals for help. Consequently, instead of spending quiet time with Nancy, I met daily with the head nurse, addressing unending concerns of Nancy's, which left me feeling overwhelmed and barely able to cope with everything rushing up at me. In addition, I had an intense fear she would be discharged and sent home, where I would be unable to care for her on my own.

The days wore on and Nancy's complaints intensified. As she became more and more angry and strident, I was increasingly unable to set my fears aside and listen to her in the manner which she deserved.

It became unpleasant to visit her. Rather than her being glad to see me, rather than her showing an understanding of how I was juggling my work schedule to visit her two and three times a day, she would bitterly complain and demand to go back to her home. At the time, it did not occur to me that this was her first stay in a nursing home. She was scared, and when she was scared, it came out as anger. I would tell her I was unable to care for her in her present condition, to please wait until she became more mobile and then she could come home. In response to my needs and suggestions, she would get angry at me. I was working so hard to do everything for her, but I was unable to handle what seemed to be anger directed at me.

At first, I did not understand that Nancy, as the patient, had to be nice to doctors and nurses. She learned quickly that if she yelled at a nurse, that person might ignore her for awhile. Accordingly, her anger and frustration were taken out on me. She knew I loved her unconditionally and I would never leave her. I was Nancy's only link to help and reality which contributed to the long list of things I had to do on her behalf.

At the end of the first week, when I went to visit Nancy, the nursing director came up to me and asked to see me in her office. I knew something was wrong but I did not know what it was. She said she was sorry to have to tell me that the day nurse had discovered a bedsore on Nancy's buttock. At this point, I could not control my anger and frustration any longer: "The care at the hospital was superb. It took only a day or two in this nursing home for Nancy to begin complaining about how people were talking to her, and how they would intentionally make her wait." The director told me she would investigate the matter. She voiced that, from her perspective, if such a problem had developed, perhaps Nancy would be better off going home or being transferred to another facility.

It was all I could do to not get upset over the implied threat of Nancy's being sent home. Due to the speed and ease with which this solution was offered to me, I suddenly sensed that the director was aware of a far larger problem.

When I went to Nancy's room, I demanded to see the bedsore. Nancy was upset and furious. She was demanding to get out of the place. Several nurses came in, rolled her over and showed me a round red angry sore the size of a silver dollar. I had never seen so clearly an open wound, with skin so red. The nurses explained that several layers of skin had been attacked and if unchecked the hole could get so deep you could put a finger in it.

I asked what caused bedsores. I was told it had to do with cleanliness and frequently moving bedridden patients from side to side. When a bedridden person lies in one position over a protracted period of time, the weight of the body causes the skin to break down. The nursing staff alluded to the fact that Nancy was a difficult patient and that she had often refused to do as instructed. They asked me how many days she had spent in the hospital prior to recently entering the nursing home.

That bedsore never healed completely. The nurses talked about its healing in time, when in actual fact, there was no way for me to know it would be there for another eighteen months. Like an old war injury, it would stay with her to her dying day.

Shortly thereafter, Nancy's unhappiness necessitated a transfer to another nursing home. I got in touch with our HMO and discovered available alternatives. There was a nursing home in the area which had just established an oncological unit. The nurses were licensed and certified to take care of cancer patients. It sounded ideal. This time I was determined to tour and approve the facility before Nancy was transferred.

The nursing home seemed eager to admit their first cancer patient. They showed me what would be her room, number one hundred and seventy-five, all the way at the end of the hall. It would be quiet. She would be alone in a double room until another cancer patient was admitted. There was a multifunctional meeting and sitting room just across the hall.

Once she was settled in, memory loss continued to be a problem. One evening, during my third visit of the day, I was flabbergasted when Nancy, all agitated, yelled out at me, "Where have you been? I've been here in this hospital bed for days waiting for you and you never showed up. You dumped me here and left me all alone."

I was absolutely frightened and heart-broken. I was exhausted, burning myself out and this was my reward!

This is where the expertise of the oncological nurses came into play. They understood what was going on and immediately told Nancy I had been there earlier. Then when Nancy would get upset over the fact that she could not remember, they were skilled in handling her crying. They consoled her and helped her. They also took me aside and told me to bring in photos of Margaux and me, preferably with Nancy. We mounted them on colorful construction paper and in big script signed them at the bottom, saying we had been there to see her. In the future, when Nancy complained about our not being there, they would point to the photos and remind her we had just been there.

Later on I was to learn that these symptoms also appear in Alzheimer's patients. Unknown to me, and working independently at the same time but many miles apart, Lorna, was busy posting similar signs and photos in the room of her father, John, who was suffering from Alzheimer's. As her father had always been intrigued with maps, she had a posted a colored and enlarged road map, with large, brightly painted homemade signs, showing exactly where he and his three children, Lorna, Murray and Aileen resided. Lorna had dreamed up this room décor for her father, as he, suffering from Alzheimer's, often became confused and disoriented due to short term memory loss, just as my Nancy did.

Margaux, too, had an experience which involved her mother's memory loss and would remain with her as one of the worst memories of her mother. While Nancy was in the second nursing home, Margaux and a friend had come to visit and Nancy had requested her favorite face cream. This extremely expensive salve came in a small jar because it was meant to be applied very sparingly to the face. Nancy opened the jar, scooped out a huge gob and started rubbing it on her hands. Margaux said, "Mom! What are you doing?"

"I don't know," Nancy said, confused. She did not

understand the question. Margaux recalls the situation, "She kept on rubbing her hands. She looked at me and it was the scariest thing. It was so sad. She was like a little kid. She had a silly childlike smile on her face." Margaux adds, "When you catch them in that moment, there's just something in their eyes that's so sad. They don't know what they are doing, as if I had caught a little kid peeing in her pants."

When loved ones do irrational things, you may feel uncomfortable and nervous. Afterwards you may feel bad you had an inappropriate response. In Margaux's case, she felt she acted stupidly.

Another disconcerting problem you will encounter is keeping track of visitors. Often when I would come into her room, I would observe flowers and gifts, and I would wonder who had visited Nancy. I knew all too well, at times she would be sleeping and it was best not to disturb her. Then, too, even when awake, she was often unable to recall who had been there. To ask her questions made matters worse because she would get angry and upset over her own forgetfulness. Consequently, Margaux and I devised a guest book.

We posted a request for people to sign their name, and the date and time they came to visit. Under such circumstances, it's not up to the patient to keep track of visitors and gifts. While we encountered limited success, again, my friend, Lorna, posted really large, colorful signs, asking visitors of her dad, to please write in her dad's "daily memory book". She also asked the nursing staff to encourage visitors' participation in her absence and to please take the time to read short excerpts to John now and then to remind him how much he was loved.

In time, Nancy's overall decline, physical collapse and memory loss combined to make her incontinent and she rightfully resented not being able to go to the bathroom on her own, when she needed to. Unable to stand on her own feet, she was dependent on nurses and orderlies when she rang for assistance. Not remembering ringing the nurses' bell or going to the bathroom, added to the confusion. Soon the nursing home started dressing her in diapers. The impact on me, seeing the mother of my child, my lover and soul mate, in diapers, was extremely disquieting.

Nancy also became neutropenic. Her blood cells had been so decimated by the toxic chemicals that she was extremely susceptible to contracting illnesses from visitors. Signs were posted at her door. I was required to wash my hands every time I came in. No flowers were allowed in the room.

Then she required a blood transfusion. An ambulance took her to the hospital to do this on an out-patient basis. With all the attention in the press about AIDS and the blood supply, when Nancy did recover and came home, there was some concern on my part about the blood she had received. If only I had thought about this earlier. If only I had planned for this contingency, perhaps I could have organized a small group of friends, with Nancy's blood type, and built up a store of compatible blood for Nancy's use.

This leads to another important point. Already exhausted between visiting her, and after putting out fires and commuting to work, I always came home to numerous messages on the answering machine. I felt too tired to listen to them, let alone make calls. However, it was an inescapable fact that if I spent an hour or so every evening calling neighbors, family and friends, and thanking them for support, or simply keeping them informed as to how Nancy was doing, I always saw an increase in her calls and visitors over the next few days. Fortunately, Nancy never really knew how hard I worked to give her these gifts.

As Nancy worked her way through therapy and started to make progress, we were able to have more fun. Increasingly she would be in the wheelchair when I arrived, not flat out on her back. One time I came to visit and she greeted me at the nurses' station. It was exhilarating to see her learning to use the rolling walker.

I started bringing in picnic fare. I would load up a basket with take-out from our favorite Italian restaurant, "Anthony's", a candle, a bottle of wine from our homemade collection and, a white rose, hand picked from a vine beside our house. We would go into the little reception room across the hall and she would enjoy the food and my company. Several nurses would come by and tell Nancy they wished their boyfriends or husbands would treat them like that. Nancy's face would beam with joy and happiness. I enjoyed the blessing of being able to return to some of our cherished rituals. In some respects, it was typical of the way we constantly worked to find the smallest window of opportunity and turn it into something pleasurable.

Nancy continued to have numerous scans and tests and there was always a problem finding a suitable vein. One radiation group collapsed the only good vein she had. As her left hand could not be used because of both the edema and removal of lymph nodes, the doctors impressed upon her the urgency to have a port installed. The procedure would be performed by the woman surgeon we both admired. On the day of the surgery Nancy insisted I go to the local jeweler to pick up the rosary which was being repaired for her. I wanted to stay in the waiting room. She demanded I go. I took about an hour to run her errand.

When I returned to the surgical waiting room, I immediately went to the volunteer receptionist and asked about the status of Nancy's surgery. The lady seemed flustered and asked me to wait. I sat down and tried to read a magazine. After about fifteen minutes I thought enough was enough. I went back to the same receptionist and asked again where Nancy was. The lady replied she had been calling around and no one knew.

I lost it. This was unconscionable. Supposedly she was in surgery or in the recovery room, yet, no one knew where she was! I told the volunteer this was unacceptable and "I would go find her myself. Thanks anyway." The volunteer panicked and told me she would page the surgeon.

The doctor showed up in about ten minutes. I then learned that Nancy had suffered some form of seizure or irregular heart beat and they were therefore unable to operate. She had been examined by the cardiologists and was waiting to be admitted to the cardiac unit for overnight observation. The news was like an electric shock coursing through my body. She could have died on a stretcher and I was out there at the jewelers. I demanded to be taken to her.

Nancy was on a stretcher in a hallway, happy to see me and able to speak. She went on to describe a chest pain she had experienced while waiting for her operation. Then everyone seemed to get excited and all these heart doctors showed up. The good news was there no longer seemed to be a problem.

I told her, in a nice and gentle, but firm manner, that this was the last time I would go anywhere when she was waiting for surgery. She was delighted to have the rosary and she promised to never send me away again under circumstances such as this.

I characterize this stage of my life as my "ambulance chasing days." It's hard to believe that I actually became accustomed to arriving at the nursing home, only to find Nancy's room empty, and upon inquiry, learn that she had been ambulanced to a hospital. Blood transfusions. Neurological examinations. Anything and everything.

Nonetheless, no matter how bad things got, there was always something good that came from it. I learned every back road, shortcut and connecting road in several counties. Without fail, I got up at five a.m. and visited her in the early morning in the nursing home or hospital. Then I commuted into the city and struggled to keep my job. Depending where she was, I would stop by to see her on the way home and I would visit with her again each evening, my third visit of the day.

While Nancy was in the nursing home, one visit with her in particular, affected me deeply. I had phoned just prior to my visit and Nancy then told me to bring cash,

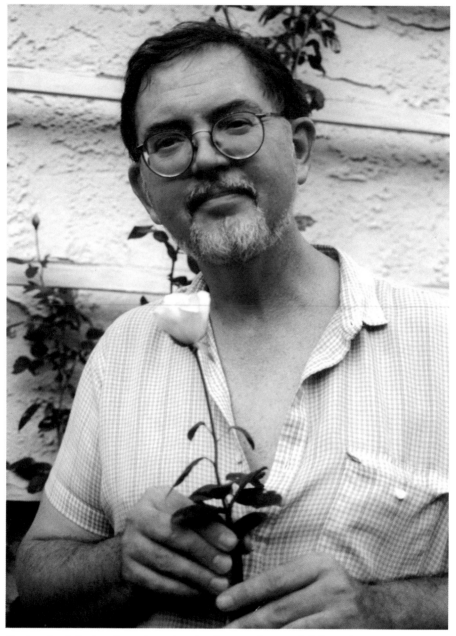

I started bringing in picnic fare. I would load up a basket with take-out from our favorite Italian restaurant, "Anthony's", a candle, a bottle of wine from our homemade collection and, a white rose, hand picked from a bush beside our house.

lots of cash. They were having a sale in the community room. When I arrived at the home, I helped her into a wheelchair and rolled her down the corridor. Nancy cheerfully informed the nurses that she was going shopping. When we got there, it reminded me of a street market. There were racks of dresses, shorts and tops and tables piled high with socks and underwear. Shoes. Bras. Anything and everything. Nancy was really enjoying herself. She selected certain garments and asked me what I thought of them. It was mind-boggling observing my loved one who had shopped Saks, Bonwits and Bloomingdale's, now getting her jollies at a nursing home's bazaar.

Easter approached and after Margaux and Nancy spent all day Saturday decorating her room, Nancy won an award. Again, I was stressed out and struggling. That Friday I had gone into work in town and had purchased special Easter candy for the three of us, as well as Nancy's siblings, who lived out of town. Returning home, I had carefully placed the white shopping bag, filled with these Easter treats, on the overhead rack of my commuter train. However, after having gotten off at my stop, I suddenly realized that I had left the candy on the train. Nancy was expecting to wrap the packages for mailing that night. There was no way to go back into town, buy new candy and get to the nursing home on time. I was heartbroken, stressed and frazzled. Frantically, I called the stationmaster, who radioed the train, which was now miles away. Later, thanks to the stationmaster's help, I went back to the train station and retrieved the candy, safe and sound. Consequently, by the time I made it to the nursing home that night, I was ready to collapse, not to wrap packages. Nancy got angry with me for not showing enthusiasm over something as important as this. She had spent all day waiting to see me and do this activity and I was spoiling it for her.

Easter Sunday, however, was a very special day. As Nancy was making such wonderful progress, I got permission to take her out of the nursing home for the day. Suzanne, our good friend and a registered nurse, offered to help. Borrowing the nursing home's wheelchair, we went to church for Easter service. We pushed Nancy in the wheelchair up the ramp to the front of the church where there were several wheelchairs in a wide handicapped area. At mass we cried. Then we went home for a rest. It was the weirdest experience, sitting in the living room from which Nancy had been absent for over two months. It was also bizarre she was in a wheelchair.

Nancy wanted to see her house so I supported her and she walked slowly from room to room. Then we sat in the living room and she questioned Margaux closely about her schoolwork and her grades for the semester.

We had reservations at a local steak house for three o'clock and Nancy insisted on taking the wheelchair over to the salad bar and picking her own ingredients. On the way home I went down a local road and I slowed to a crawl for all of us to soak in an incredibly beautiful sight. For about half a mile, as far around the bend as the eye could see, there was a breathtaking row of flowering fruit trees in full bloom. As the trees were all large and the same size, the whiteness of the display was not only dazzling, but also comforting and uplifting.

Back home once again, Nancy wanted to lie down in our bed for a rest. She expressed how restrictive and uncomfortable hospital beds were and how it felt so good to be in her own bed once again. I lay on one side of Nancy and Margaux lay on the other. The three gummy bears were reunited again. None of us slept, but the silence was profound. We each were processing our own thoughts. Consequently, at the end of the day, it was incredibly sad taking Nancy back to the nursing home.

Nancy applied herself to physical therapy and after Easter she came home. Then the visits to the oncologist became a regular feature in our lives. Nancy and I had to go every other week without fail, morning or afternoon, Monday through Friday, to receive her chemotherapy. In those days, evening and weekend treatment hours were unheard of in this specialized field.

The potential side effects of these powerful treatments can be devastating and life threatening. As Nancy underwent extensive testing, it was discovered the decadron had made her diabetic. Over the years her blood sugar levels had already tested in the high end of the range. Now her sugar levels were totally out of control. She was put on insulin and we were assured, after the decadron levels were reduced, her blood sugar levels would come down. What they didn't tell us was that it would take quite a while to bring this condition under control.

I have always had an aversion to needles. While Nancy was in the nursing home, there were always nurses to give her an injection. However, when she was sent home, this became a significant problem as Nancy was unable to administer the drug to herself. The health plan then insisted I should learn to give her the daily injection which I simply was unable to do. Fortunately, once again, Suzanne offered to help. She stopped over daily and gave Nancy her injection.

As Nancy's chemotherapy progressed, it took a cumulative toll, reducing her white blood cell count to dangerous levels. Her oncologist then prescribed a drug which would restore her white blood cells. From there on, a different routine emerged at the pharmacy, as the druggist stated it would take a few days to get the prescription filled in the store. Apparently it was a relatively new drug and it was extremely expensive. Therefore it was not kept in stock. When I questioned how expensive the new drug would be, I was told that a dozen vials would retail for about $2,500. Luckily, at that time, my insurance had a co-pay of just $5. When the medicine came, Nancy held it in her hands with an awestruck expression on her face. I think it drove home the severity of her situation. She was in uncharted waters. Even the Zofran which would combat her nausea was extremely expensive. This financial

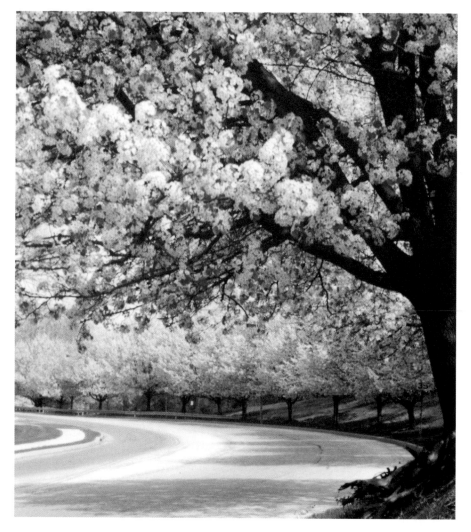

For about half a mile, as far around the bend as the eye could see, there was a breathtaking row of flowering fruit trees in full bloom. As the trees were all large and the same size, the whiteness of the display was not only dazzling, but also comforting and uplifting.

escalation exemplified the levels to which the battle had intensified.

I was stunned by the domino effect. One medication or treatment triggered negative side effects, leading to even more medications, which led to other medications. I was gravely concerned about the cumulative, long term effect. I also realized, if I had not had insurance, or had the plan been less comprehensive, it would have been financially crippling to pay for these unending treatments.

The routine for Nancy's chemotherapy looked like this. I routinely scheduled a half-day off from work to drive her. We checked in and presented her referral. Next we went to the basement where she had blood drawn. We then took the elevator back up and sat in the waiting room until we were called. In the examining room Nancy changed into a gown and we waited again. The blood counts were important. The oncologist was basically trying to inject as high a dose of chemo as possible. If the counts were too low, he could not inject any more drugs. If they were moderate, he could increase the dosage.

Nancy's port was under the skin on her right upper chest wall. Once or twice she received chemo sitting up and complained of the odor. We consequently learned it was best for her to lie down.

For me, juggling my business schedule was a constant struggle. We tried to schedule appointments early in the morning or late in the afternoon. With forgetfulness being a major issue, my role, in addition to vigilance and support, was to be the custodian of her long list of questions and the scribe of each and every response. Nancy had zero tolerance if I missed recording a white or red blood count. For days afterwards, we would repeatedly discuss what was said, as she could often not remember and my notations served to help her process and come to decisions.

From there on, our problems increased. For example, one day she pointed to her eye and asked me what I thought. Taking time to observe carefully, I commented that the left eye appeared to be a trifle droopy. I observed that perhaps she was tired. Nancy burst out in anger that it had been that way for days. Then she broke down and cried. I hugged her and comforted her. As far as Nancy was concerned, it had to be cancer. First Nancy discussed it with her oncologist. She was determined to really find out what it was. This triggered another series of doctors' visits.

First, we went to the primary physician for a referral. Then, we consulted with a neurological specialist. Finally, we sought a second opinion and discovered it was Horner's Disease, which could be caused by a small tumor somewhere on the nerve running from the brain to the eye. There was no way to find such a small tumor, but, hopefully the chemotherapy would shrink it and her eye might get better. It never did. She suffered from this condition to the day she died.

Even though Nancy's physical condition was rapidly deteriorating, all was not doom and gloom. Around this time, my first book was published and copies started rolling off the presses. For me, this represented a dream come true. For Nancy, it was something positive to embrace and enjoy. I remember her saying to a friend on the phone, "We talk about more than cancer in this household! Let me tell you about Anthony's book."

One ongoing major issue for supportive care providers is how to balance work and family obligations. During the intense phase of Nancy's fight I had an understanding manager, Pete, who would do just about anything to help me through each crisis. One of the most important things he did was to have the courage to ask me how things were going and this he did over and over again. I was extremely emotional at this time and thus when I responded to his questions, uncontrollable tears often accompanied my answer, which this boss had the courage to handle. I always knew he cared.

His interest and support transcended what must have been an extraordinarily difficult incident for him. The bank was in a nine month exercise of eliminating thousands of jobs and Nancy came to see the bank as the devil and my boss as the devil's accomplice. Consequently, one day, while hallucinating, Nancy ranted and raved against the bank and my boss and, over my objections, she picked up the phone, called my boss and heaped venom and anger on him. I was flabbergasted. Here was the person who was going out of his way to help me and he was dumped upon.

The next day at work, my manager was visibly shaken, but supportive and understanding. Over the long haul I learned he never let that incident bother him. He was a big person indeed to understand it was Nancy's illness, not the person, Nancy, who had been speaking on the phone the previous day. Possibly, he felt empathy for me having to face that on a daily basis.

However, during the final phase of Nancy's illness I also experienced the exact opposite. I then had a boss who did not want to know anything about Nancy's problems. When I needed time off, she followed company policy to the letter, no more, no less. She also made it clear that there were others in the department with serious family problems, that I was not alone. She could not treat me any differently than the others. Her position felt hard and uncaring.

Thus I encountered both extremes and was grateful for any help I received. In our stressful, busy, highly competitive work environment, it's difficult for a manager to extend help in crisis situations, while keeping up the pace of a department's workload.

Happily, some companies are recognizing the human side of doing business by introducing enlightened policies and procedures in the workplace. One such story, as reported in the Wall Street Journal, involves Bill Foote, CEO of USG Corporation. Shortly after his wife's diagnosis of breast cancer, he told his managers at a meeting that his family was "facing one of the biggest challenges we're ever going to face, and I'm going to need some help." His 42-year-old wife, Andrea, succumbed to the illness fourteen months later, after an intense battle. A private person by nature, Mr. Foote broke precedent by openly talking about his grief and the new role of being a single parent with three daughters, aged thirteen, eleven and ten. He opened his first speech as CEO to one hundred and fifty managers by telling them that life is precious and fleeting. "Live in the moment. Simplify your days to emphasize what really matters: kids, self, family, work. I love USG. My number one priority is my family." His statements were consistent with his management philosophy of engaging the total self in the workplace: he valued teamwork, trust, openness and honesty about weaknesses, as well as strengths.

On what was to be, unknown to us, our last Christmas, I was able to enjoy time off for the Holidays. Around this time Nancy had a powerful dream.

"Pocahontas. It was a Pocahontas dream," Nancy said.

Not being a swimmer, I was at a total loss as to what Pocahontas meant. "What does Pocahontas mean?"

"It's rhythm, treading water. Staying alive."

"How did it feel?"

"I felt very skinny. I was naked, in a backyard pool. I did not want to be Pocahontas. I was too skinny. Besides, it was not my property."

I wondered why it was a backyard pool when it could have been an ocean or a lake. Nancy had often talked about almost drowning in Lake Erie when she was young.

After her death, the possible significance of this dream became clearer to me. The controlled environment was the radiation and the chemotherapy. All it was doing was keeping her alive. She was getting nowhere. The nausea and side-effects of chemotherapy had caused an undesired weight loss which troubled her deeply.

The telling of this dream had a profound effect on Margaux and she expressed her feelings in a painting. Interestingly, the swimmer in the painting looked like

Margaux, not Nancy. (At Nancy's viewing, we displayed a dramatic black and white photograph, a head shot of Nancy as a young woman. Everyone thought it was a photograph of Margaux.)

When told she had three to four months to live because her cancer had spread to major organs, Nancy often wondered aloud, "Am I living or am I dying?" Reality becomes a fine line for the terminally ill. Here's what worked for us. I would ask her, "Can you see this beautiful day? Are you enjoying it?" She would answer affirmatively and I would conclude, "Clearly, you are living! It is the essence of life to enjoy a beautiful day." On a personal level, this ongoing exchange was easier for me to handle than casting her clumps of chemo-stricken hair to the winds.

As Nancy's battle became increasingly desperate, the temptation to explore fringe therapies became stronger. She showed an intense interest in news articles about physicians experimenting with different drugs, megadoses of medications and herbs, and unproven techniques.

This approach again put me in a difficult position. Part of me wanted to be positive and supportive. Who would want to deprive someone with no prospects, of any opportunity to find a cure or to prolong life? However, another side of me saw these experimental therapies for what they were; risky procedures outside accepted practices, taking huge risks in an attempt to make a breakthrough. One doctor specializing in medicinal mega-doses was interviewed with one or two patients who had experienced success. The end of the article was an interview with a person who had lost a loved one to the treatment. Fortunately, Nancy made up her own mind, first considering, then rejecting such alternatives, based on her own observations. Numerous others, however, become emotionally and financially bankrupt while pursuing similar experimental therapies.

Another major issue was the dispensing of her numerous medications. Taking into account her short

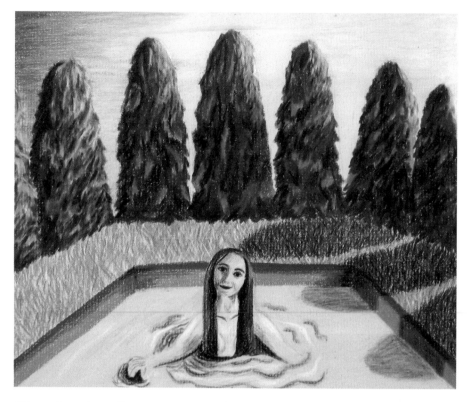

"*Pocahontas. It was a Pocahontas dream,*" Nancy said. *Not being a swimmer, I was at a total loss as to what Pocahontas meant. "It's rhythm, treading water. Staying alive," said Nancy.*

term memory loss, she took the initiative to devise a system for making sure she took all her pills each day establishing a designated place in the kitchen. Each morning she counted out all her pills and put them in a plastic bowl. Depending on how much medication she was taking at any point in time, she would write out the sequence of pills for the day. For the most part, Nancy managed the process for herself. However, it is often the case that this job needs to be supervised by, and in time, becomes the responsibility of the caretaker.

One Sunday when we got up we were greeted by a steady soaking rain. It was a happy rain after weeks of hot sunny days. Several communities had already initiated drought restrictions. The sky alternated patches of bright blue with large fast-moving rain clouds.

In Church, I observed that Nancy was emotional. She started to cry. She whispered to me that she felt a sadness. Not a depression, but a sadness. I asked if there was anything specific. She said, "No." After Mass, she went out the main aisle, not the side entrance by which we had come in. I assumed she wanted to chat with several of our friends. She always drew energy from people.

Driving home, she started crying again. I offered to pull over and talk. She wanted to go home. As we drove, we talked and she cried. At a stop light, a dead butterfly fell from the sun visor or blew up from the air vent. The two of us stared at it incredulously! Butterflies had been her friends, following her all summer and fall and a dear friend had given her a butterfly window hanging. Even her support group had autographed the back of a butterfly shirt for her. And here, now, we stared at this dead butterfly. I took a tissue to pick it up and throw it out later. Nancy said, "Maybe it's still alive. Maybe we could let it go on the lawn and see if it will live." As I wrapped up the tissue, I said it was definitely dead. Later that day I thought about that moment and experienced regret and anxiety over being such a clod. Several months after she died, I realized that Nancy had made a transition from cherishing free fluttering butterflies to focusing on angels around this time. Nancy had also gone back to our practice of scattering her hair over the lawn, to come back another day. What a nice way to substitute something positive for the pain of the moment. And, I was unable to pick up on it.

When we got home, we sat on the sofa and I asked her to talk about the sadness, to please describe it. She talked about seeing a close friend at the support group meeting on Thursday. How good she looked. Her hair had grown back and she had it cut very short and looked like a cute pixie. I recalled we had seen her at the doctor's the last time Nancy had had chemotherapy. "She's having radiation to the legs for bone cancer," Nancy explained, and then broke down sobbing.

I asked if she was sad over the fear of recurrence? The fear of when and how her cancer would come back swept over the two of us and we cried together. Nancy also talked about her fatigue over carrying on with the fight. No matter how hard she fought, no matter how far she came, cancer was always there doggedly following her.

That afternoon we went to a movie, a comedy. Three guys in drag. That same day we prayed, cried and laughed together. Not since February had I felt death looking in my windows. Death was stalking us again. I felt an overwhelming fear for our future. I felt the intensity of work and a sense of inadequacy to handle the two. Would I crash this time? How much would she suffer when it came back?

Speaking of the future, little did I know that after Nancy died there would be one single thing which could have made a big difference for Margaux and me. We both missed the sight of her, we missed her hugs, and, above all, we missed the sound of her voice. In a moment of desperation, Margaux said, "I'd give anything to hear mom's voice, just one more time. Even if she was angry and yelling at me." Then too, shortly after Nancy's death,

I dreamed I had found an answering machine with her voice saying 'Hi Boo! Love 'ya. Angel.' This was a happy dream. I was delighted to unexpectedly find a tape and hear her voice again.

When Nancy was on her extended course of chemotherapy, my position at the bank was eliminated. Miraculously, I quickly landed a job with a leading firm in our area. As I was anxious to celebrate, and sensing we had little time, I quickly worked the yellow pages and called every inn, motel and bed and breakfast in Cape May, New Jersey. Nancy kept talking about Cape Cod, but Margaux and I both agreed that Nancy was too weak for a trip of that magnitude. We therefore picked Cape May based on Nancy's loving the shops and the fact that it was closer to home.

Once there, Margaux and I went fishing. It was my lucky day as I reeled in one fish after another. I wound up splitting the boat's wagering pool as one of my flounders was tied for the largest fish. It felt marvelous after all the ongoing stresses, tensions, and exhausting timetables.

Although the three of us had agreed earlier that Nancy did not want to go fishing, and for physical reasons should not go, when Margaux and I returned to the motel room, Nancy voiced strong regrets about not having gone. We smoothed it over, but the palpable feeling in the room was that she sensed it was her last chance to go on a boat and to see her loved ones fish. It was so sad and melancholy that in only a moment or two, I went from joy to depression. Five months after she died, I still felt overwhelmed by the sadness of this memory, and I could not hold back the tears.

On the way back from this vacation, I spontaneously suggested we go to Atlantic City. Nancy loved to play the slots. She had seemed a trifle down on the Garden State Parkway and this perked her up. In life there are certain images of extreme happiness and joy so intense they sear themselves into the cells of your brain; Nancy at the slots, so weak she could hardly stand up, yet energized and invigorated, pumping quarters into a machine. Happiness beamed from her countenance.

It felt good to give her so much pleasure. Then, I noticed a flashing button on the slot machine. I pressed it and good-luck quarters tumbled into the tray. Suddenly I realized Nancy's mind was totally disconnected from the activity. She had not focused on the flashing light. Was this her brain tumor robbing her of memory and consciousness once again? In a flash I experienced a profound sense of depression.

Now here's what you can do.....

* Approach and accept your family and friends as a critical support network. Perhaps you can find a friend who would be willing to keep other close friends caught up on your loved one's progress, on your behalf, via emails or a chain phone calling arrangement. This, in turn, could help decrease the time you spend updating friends in general and increase the much needed time and energy you have for your loved one. A friend's scheduling rides, by volunteers, for your loved one, may also be needed and appreciated. It may even be possible to obtain volunteers who are willing to donate the precious gift of a compatible blood supply for your loved one.
* Recognize the tremendous responsibility which falls upon the family caring for and supporting someone with a history of cancer. How could we have known that forgetfulness was a major clue of her evolving brain tumor? Why did her medical team not give us a checklist of signs and symptoms of things to look for? Why did specialists not listen to, hear and respond to my persistent statements that something was wrong? The burden of responsibility, as a caring, loving partner, requires you to go out of your way to observe and note anything out of the ordinary.

* You must be assertive, discussing your observations with your loved ones and the doctors. You must be open to your own inner voice or intuition, which will tell you when something is truly wrong. It's not an easy task, but it is a gift of inestimable value to the person who, for a variety of reasons, may very well be incapable of self-monitoring.

* Not only are health benefits of prime concern to you, care must be taken regarding prescription plans. For example, some require a five dollar or ten dollar co-pay with each filled prescription. Under such circumstances ask your doctors to prescribe as large a quantity as possible. Health insurers will draw a line but you need to push to find out just where that line is.

* Other plans can require you to pay as much as fifty per cent of the cost of each prescription. It is difficult to foresee, yet, such a plan can pose economic hardship when dealing with expensive, newly approved, leading-edge drugs.

* Consider contributing to your local volunteer ambulance corps. In turn, take advantage of their support should an emergency trip to the hospital be required.

* While many people tend to be private about personal life crises and losses in the workplace, there is a new spirit of openness. If talking about things works for you, try it at work. Be aware that some folks will respond warmly and supportively. Others will be unable to engage in dialogue. Accept each response unconditionally.

* Consider informing your manager about what is going on in your life. Again, it is a matter of individual judgment to determine the level of detail your manager is ready, willing, or able to handle.

* If you are a manager in a crisis situation, you have a tremendous opportunity to make an empathetic difference.

* Take into consideration the fact that the ill person may not always say what is really on his or her mind. This may be an avoidance/coping mechanism resulting from

fear, hurt and pain.

* There are precious rare moments when it is good to cry together. Choose these moments carefully, assessing the impact on the other person. Breast cancer survivors carry substantial baggage over guilt: guilt over getting sick, guilt over stressing and burdening their families, guilt over loss of income and fear that medical expenses may cause severe financial losses.

* If required to select a nursing home, try to visit as many as possible in advance. Do not blame yourself if you are unable to take care of your loved one's physical and emotional needs within your home setting, but do try and include your loved one in the nursing home tours and subsequent decisions as often as is practically possible.

* Be prepared to sign an imposing and overwhelming stack of forms. Before signing however, be careful that legal technicalities are fully explained to your satisfaction.

* Talk to friends, neighbors and clergy to gather information about nursing homes in your area, thus obtaining relatively dependable opinions, concerning the quality of care provided. For example, the clergy at a local church probably spend several hours a week visiting the sick. They therefore have their own first hand impressions of the facilities in your area. As they listen to the patients in these facilities, they can refer you to family members of patients for more first hand information. Furthermore, they may also know which facilities have specialized units, specifically suited to your loved one's illness.

* Take time to identify your individual needs and requirements as well as your loved one's. For example, ask insurance carriers if exceptions can be made when something such as counseling for you is not typically covered.

* Inquire about specialized oncological or Alzheimer's units in nursing homes. Follow up with questions about the credentials of the nursing staff. Are their specialized

skills aligned with the types of patient in the unit where they work?

* It would help their loved ones immensely if terminally ill people left something behind. It could possibly be a written letter or an audio taped message. It need not be original. A mother could read an article or poem with special meaning to a beloved daughter, son or perhaps even a grandchild. The more ambitious could video-tape a message and record their image. However, women suffering with breast cancer and hair loss might reject this possibility. This could also be a viable alternative for someone in the very early stages of Alzheimer's. Loving care providers can be helpful in raising the subject, suggesting, perhaps even asking the ill person to consider leaving something personal behind.

CHAPTER 6
Final Stages

"Learn to detach....But detachment doesn't mean you don't let the experience penetrate you. On the contrary, you let it penetrate you fully. That's how you are able to leave it....Take any emotion-love for a woman, or grief for a loved one, or what I'm going through, fear and pain from a deadly illness. If you hold back on the emotions – if you don't allow yourself to go all the way through them – you can never get to being detached, you're too busy being afraid. You're afraid of the pain, you're afraid of the grief. You're afraid of the vulnerability that loving entails. But by throwing yourself into these emotions, by allowing yourself to dive in, all the way, over your head even, you experience them fully and completely. You know what pain is. You know what love is. You know what grief is. And only then can you say, 'All right. I have experienced that emotion. I recognize that emotion. Now I need to detach from that emotion for a moment'....When you learn how to die, you learn how to live."

These are the words of Morrie Schwartz, a college professor, spoken when he knew he was dying of amyotrophic lateral sclerosis (ALS), also known as Lou Gehrig's disease. *Tuesdays with Morrie* by Mitch Albom.

It is said that the shadowy world of dreams is where our subconscious has the greatest freedom of expression. Watching a person die and helping them prepare for death, is an experience of reality which many liken to the unreality of a deep dream.

At the end, there is a total lack of clarity as to when death will occur. You are pre-occupied with living in the moment, struggling to ensure quality care, possibly trying to keep up with a job and perhaps with children, plus constantly worrying about financial matters. These things all distract from the real issue at hand.

There is also an eerie unknown timetable in the final stages. I'll never forget the winter Nancy's physician said she had three to four months to live. She lived for eighteen months. Then, when I was told she had two months to live, she lived only two weeks. But, I am getting ahead of myself.

During the Spring of 1996, my position was eliminated in a bank merger. I was out of work and my wife was dying. I was not surprised by the hard boss who showed no empathy. Instantly I forgave her, refusing to allow anger or resentment into my heart. However, I did feel at a disadvantage in my job search. Other candidates were free to entertain offers wherever they pleased. I felt tied to my existing HMO, and consequently, geographically restricted in my search.

Miraculously, I found a good job in less than three months. It was closer to home than I had ever been. Most importantly, my new employer offered the same health care coverage.

At that time I had mixed feelings about this stroke of good fortune. Ideally, in a fantasy world, I would rather have used the opportunity to go into business for myself. However, in our present predicament, this was entirely out of the question, as continuity of health care benefits was our number one agenda item. Any discrepancy with pre-existing conditions meant certain financial ruin. The pressures I felt were intense, bordering upon debilitating.

Once I secured this much needed job, Nancy started focusing on her own issues. She initiated conversations about walking away from treatment. She felt exhaustion of mind, body and spirit. She had received fifteen months of chemotherapy which was holding the cancer in abeyance, but not pushing it back. Now she often required a wheelchair to get around.

The presence of the wheelchair freaked me out. It was painful to see her weakened to the point she could not walk. As I also suffered from chronic back pain, pushing a wheelchair up an inclined handicap ramp often strained my lower back muscles.

Even more painful was the 14th of July, when Nancy asked to have a family discussion. It was late one dark, stormy, steamy Saturday afternoon. Nancy, Margaux and I sat in our living room on the white sofa we had so carefully selected fifteen years earlier. We called ourselves the 'three gummy bears.' It must have been absolutely bizarre for Nancy and Margaux as I started out the discussion talking about treatment options. I soon sensed that they really wanted to talk about something else.

Margaux opened things up when she said, "Mom, I support you no matter what you decide to do. If you want to walk away from treatment, it's okay. I've tried to put myself in your position and I don't know if I would have been able to take as much as you have." Nancy jumped right in, crying, saying that Margaux heard her and understood how she felt. There was a massive three-way cleansing cry.

My head was spinning. I realized in a flash that I had missed the point altogether. To a degree, I felt left out. They were comfortable talking about this, whereas I was struggling. The end of Nancy's life flashed in front of my eyes. She was going to walk away from treatment and the cancer would spread through her body, unchecked and unchallenged.

Nancy talked of her pain and her frustrations. Margaux said she wanted her mother to die with dignity, her head held high. We talked about last night's pork chop dinner. Nancy had been embarrassed. She had wanted another pork chop but she was too exhausted to cut it up for herself and she had not wanted to ask for help. When I had noticed her hesitation and offered to get it for her, she was touched; profoundly moved and profoundly embarrassed at the same time. She called me her "loving matte", so obviously enjoying helping her. Yet, she was clear—she did not want to live that way.

She talked about her fears regarding her leg pains. She was fearful she would not be able to walk. She felt it was an omen that a close friend developed similar pains just before she died from cancer. She could not believe the exhaustion. There was no way she would go on Taxol, as recommended. This conversation about walking away from treatment continued to be very uncomfortable for me. I was struggling inside myself, struggling big time.

Nancy framed it in a positive light. God had not answered her prayer for a cure. Perhaps God was testing the strength of her faith. Maybe, when she gave up treatment, He would cure her Himself. If not, He would surely take her up to Heaven. I was quick to note this was the classic win/win situation. No way she could lose. That was what I said. However, what I felt was a terrifying fear of losing her and of the cancer raging unchecked. I didn't want to give her up, even if it meant her going to Heaven. I felt I couldn't tell her this; I did not want to disrupt her positive frame of mind. I faulted myself for being so slow to let go of all of my assumptions and pre-conceptions......and of her.

Margaux was reassuring. It was all right to refuse treatment if it was no longer helping her mom, but instead was tiring her and weakening her, to the point she could not enjoy living.

Nancy was quick to point out she had a tremendous desire to live. She had been carrying this burden for weeks and she did not know how to talk about it without hurting someone. I knew that someone was me. Talking about it gave her relief that she had options. Options other than unending and debilitating chemotherapy, that in the end left her in a place she definitely did not want to be.

Her skin cancer had not healed after more than six months of treatment. Now she also suffered a stress fracture. She hated what all of this was doing to her body and she was frustrated not being able to move. Her greatest fear was being kept alive without being able to "live".

Margaux was relieved to get the subject out on the table. I broke down, sobbing. I could not let go and move forward. I admitted it was my problem. I was embarrassed I found it so hard to face this issue. Margaux said it was because Nancy and I were soul-mates for so long.

Then Margaux talked about her greatest fear. She sobbed and shared with us that she was afraid of being alone in the world with no one. She admitted she had friends, but no one could replace her mom and dad. Nancy reinforced the unconditional nature of our love. I talked about confidence and inner strength. Nancy said we would always be there for Margaux, even if we were in Heaven praying for her. I stressed the need for an inner strength to live one's life according to one's convictions. To follow your star. This inner confidence could help sustain Margaux even if the two of us should die.

I then realized my greatest fear was the same as Margaux's; the fear of being left alone as an only child with no living parents.

We all agreed we had the three of us. Ourselves against the world. We did a profound, moving, three-way gummy bear hug. We pledged to be there for each other no matter what. Relief, calm and inner peace settled over the three of us and although a huge wave of exhaustion rolled over me, we kept on talking. We all felt a need to savor this wonderful moment.

Margaux then shared her determination to get a tattoo. She chose a guardian angel on her shoulder to be with her forever, to always remind her of her mom; her tremendous courage, determination and will to live.

My very close friend, George, had told me earlier that day that my new job would be my connection to the real world. My therapy. My relief. Now, Nancy said the same thing. She was so happy for me. She did not want me to be with her every moment to the end because she knew how hard that would be on me.

All of a sudden I realized Nancy knew she was dying before her doctors came to that conclusion. She walked away from treatment before they withheld her treatments.

Over what was to be the last summer of her life, I had been preoccupied with helping Nancy manage her increasingly complex health care requirements, then losing a job and finding a job. Consequently, I had little time to spend gardening or taking care of the outside of the house. As each summer storm rolled through our neighborhood and I was unable to tidy up afterwards, our five row vineyard which I had so painstakingly planted, started leaning from west to east. At first it was one vine or two, then more. Finally, near the end of the summer, it was as if some heavenly hand had pushed all the plants down to the earth. It was as if they were kneeling and praying for Nancy, waiting for her to die.

That night, I said the following prayer and came to a resolution within myself. "This is something I have no control over. We all have to die sometime. Death is absolutely inevitable. I will face this as a positive, natural experience. I can't change it. I can't influence it. It is perfectly natural. Whatever Nancy's decision, good things will come from it. My role is to support her, love her, comfort her and add as much joy and happiness to her life as I can, no matter what happens."

"Dear God, I now understand the meaning of the phrase, 'Thy will be done.' I understand thoroughly that Christ suffered mightily to save us all. I understand thoroughly that suffering can be the road to salvation and it can be positively offered up to you. But dear Lord, she has suffered enough. Please spare her and bring her up to your heavenly kingdom with grace and dignity and, please, with not too much more pain and suffering. Thank you God. Amen."

At that time, religion comforted me through Nancy's suffering. Now, several years later, re-reading this prayer, I am in a different place spiritually.

That July morning, Nancy was ironing, but by that night, her legs could not support her and she crumbled to the floor next to our bed. The extreme weakness of her legs continued Sunday. On Monday she went into the hospital for tests. It took four days to determine that the cancer had spread to the fluid in her spine. Several of the tests were dangerous, painful and difficult for her to tolerate. A spinal tap to obtain fluid for testing was particularly hard on her. Not only was the cancer now affecting her legs, it was seriously attacking her mind.

Nancy simply could not remember that she was in the hospital, rather than in her home. Her eyes were open and she could see she was in a hospital room, but in her mind, she was at home. She therefore wanted to go to her kitchen and she fought with me to go down the stairs to the basement to check on the laundry. She was angry and frustrated, that in her own house, she could not go into her own kitchen.

Not knowing what was going on, she continued her fight. She cajoled visitors into helping her out of bed to go to the bathroom, to look in the mirror. Anything. Any excuse to try to get out of bed and stand on her own two feet. She strongly believed that if she could not stand, it would be virtually impossible for her to maintain even a semblance of a quality of life.

The first night of being hospitalized, she talked me into walking her to the bathroom. Although she was unsteady, we made it to the commode. Just as she started to sit, all strength and energy flowed out of her legs, like water careening over the edge of Niagara Falls. I instantly reacted, instinctively and protectively, trying to hold her up. In a flash, I felt pain in my lower back and she crashed onto the toilet seat, banging her swollen arm hard into the metal safety bar. The two of us were shaken. I called for a nurse and it turned out everything was okay, but I instructed the hospital staff to keep a close eye on her. That night I also warned Margaux to no longer help her mother get out of bed.

The very next day, Margaux was visiting, and somehow Nancy talked her into just letting her stand next to the bed. She promised not to walk anywhere, just stand up for a moment. Suddenly, she lost her balance, her legs failed and she crashed into the wall, her skull making a loud cracking noise as it made contact with the hard cement.

80

At work, my phone rang and our daughter was on the line. Screaming. Hysterical. She felt it was her fault and she thought her mother had killed herself, or, at least seriously hurt her head. My life felt totally out of control. It was unreal, sitting there in a cubicle, with absolutely no privacy, while comforting and consoling Margaux, and, in time, realizing my voice had risen. Consequently, scores of associates could hear our private business and there was nothing I could do about it. I told Margaux over and over again that it was not her fault. It was the responsibility of the hospital staff. I was unable to speak with Nancy because she appeared to be out cold. Doctors and nurses were rushing into the room as I spoke with our daughter. I was extremely anxious to find out what had happened. I had to initiate a series of phone calls to get that information and to make sure it would not happen again.

Within a day or two, a chilling diagnosis was pronounced. At nine a.m. I received a call at work from the oncologist. He told me there was nothing else that could be done for Nancy and she needed to leave the hospital that day. The insurance would not cover her stay if no tests were being performed. All at once, I wanted to go visit her and to be with her. Simultaneously, I had to explain the situation to our daughter and arrange for a transfer, all in a matter of hours.

I called home and told Margaux I needed to talk with her face-to-face. Home for the summer, she was still half-asleep but she knew something significant had occurred. I told her I was coming right home, to get up and get her contacts in. Once again, I was the one who had to break the news to Margaux.

When we went to the hospital, Nancy was unaware of her situation. This upset me, but, there was no way to prove she had not been told as it was too easy to attribute this to her memory loss. Again, everything was falling on my shoulders.

In a rush, I transferred Nancy to the nursing home

and they kindly assigned her to her old room. However, this transfer was a nightmare. Even the ambulance was late. When we arrived, the person assigned to meet us had had to leave for the day and no one was aware of any of Nancy's numerous special requirements. I therefore went to the admissions office and did not return to Nancy's room until I felt I had made sure everything important was specified on her chart. That night, Margaux and I returned home, totally drained.

When I went back the next morning, Nancy was so tired, it was difficult to converse. After a good bit of effort, we had just begun to discuss several important issues, when a loud cheerful voice boomed into the room, "Good morning Mrs. Garbowski! Are you looking forward to fun activities today?" Nancy looked at her, thoroughly bewildered, and said, "I can't get out of this bed, what fun activities are you talking about?" The name tag clearly identified this individual as a volunteer, who was obviously unaware of the circumstances, and, inadvertently, had created an intrusion.

At that moment I knew this stay in the nursing home was very different. Last year Nancy was able to look forward to therapy with the hope that she could fight back. This time she was here to face death. She would be unable to come to grips with her personal terminal situation with any dignity with the overextended staff, noise and commotion. Even the simple act of securing a bedpan could be a nerve-wracking and upsetting ordeal. I made a promise to her on the spot, to get her home as soon as possible, making it clear that I first had to line up home nursing and negotiate with the insurance company.

It made me sick to my stomach to think I might not be able to pull it off. I could not even imagine I would not be able to give her this gift. And a gift it became. The last gift I was ever to give her. The first two home nursing services I contacted were unable to guarantee the around the clock coverage we needed. A third, recommended by a close friend, Linda, said it could be done but they would need at least one day to set it up. The insurance company graciously agreed to provide hospice and in addition, several hours a day of home nursing care. The remainder would be my financial responsibility.

Until our era of health care cost containment, terminally ill patients often died in the hospital. Today, hospitals discharge cancer patients, sending them home or into intermediate care facilities such as nursing homes. Typically, the decision revolves around what your insurance carrier covers. Some will pay for nursing home care.

Other insurance carriers provide hospice care at home. The role of hospice is to prepare the patient for death, while providing support for the family facing a loss. In the case of cancer, hospice is recommended when there is nothing further that can be done for the patient, when there is no longer a reasonable hope that treatment will keep the disease at bay or induce remission. Keeping the patient comfortable and free of pain is the best that can be expected.

At home or in a nursing home environment, you will be told that modern drugs will keep your loved one free of pain. However, there are important side effects which contribute to the process of the body's shutting down in preparation for death. In reality, morphine suppresses the entire organism, slowing breathing, and reducing the flow of oxygen to the brain. Then too, when a person lies in bed for several weeks, muscles deteriorate and atrophy to the point they will be unable to work on their own. As previously mentioned, bed sores are another real problem. Bed-ridden patients are also at greater risk of developing pneumonia. Chemotherapy severely compromises the immune system. In the final analysis, depending upon what parts of the body have been affected by the cancer, there is a chance even morphine may not suppress pain.

Most hospice programs provide for a nurse to visit several times a week and nurses' aides, several hours a day. However, there are significant problems for partners, who want to be partners but not nurses and bedpan changers. Furthermore, family members are often called upon to administer injections. Consequently, there is often total disregard for the caregiver's feelings and abilities and the impact such procedures may have on them, at a time when their nervous systems are already severely taxed and compromised.

Some families seek around the clock nursing aide care only to find the expense prohibitive and the availability limited or non-existent.

There are also physical and emotional issues when a patient comes home to die. Where should one place the hospital bed? In the bedroom, in the living room? One must consider both the dying and those who will be required to live in the house during the final stages. One should also be prepared for incomplete instructions on how to operate oxygen machines. The hospice instructed us not to call '911' or the police because emergency medical personnel are required by law to resuscitate dying patients. They cited examples of terminally ill cancer patients, with racking pain, being brought back to life, only to experience brain damage on top of all their other ills.

The thought of home care was of great interest to Nancy but she wanted to know how much it would cost. She indicated she would stay in the nursing home if it involved out-of-pocket expenses. Then, in the same instant, she looked deep in my eyes and told me how much she longed to see her home again. She missed its peace, quiet and familiarity.

Therefore, when I went to the nursing home to present the news to Nancy, I was concerned that the financial consequences of the arrangement would affect her decision about coming home. She had always been extremely sensitive about how much treatment she required and its potential to drain us financially.

Nancy and I now had an important decision to make.

The choice was either for her to remain in the nursing home and the insurance company would pay for everything, or, she could come home and we would have to pay for substantial nursing aid.

When Nancy asked if the insurance would cover care in the home, I told her they were very generous and would cover a portion. There would be a small sum each day, but not to worry, as it was like staying at a hotel. I also made it clear to her I wanted to be her husband and could not be her nurse. She understood completely.

Under similar circumstances, some care-givers might very well be comfortable providing nursing type care. In our case, physically, Nancy required total support. She was virtually incapacitated, needing to be lifted to get on and off the bedpan. She even needed help to be turned in the bed. In the nursing home, it took two nurses just to change her bed sheets. Physically I could not do this kind of lifting. Psychologically, I did not want to change her bedpan.

From a practical standpoint, it took a week to get her home. She arrived, exhausted, glorious and radiant, on our 27th wedding anniversary. Our very thoughtful friend and neighbor, Janice, presented us with a home made lasagna and I reached way in the back of the wine cellar to find a seventeen year old Italian Barolo. She savored small sips and small bites while confined to a hospital bed in our extra bedroom, the TV room. Once again, we transformed the most difficult of moments into a celebration of life and love.

No sooner had I gotten her home and made her as comfortable as could be, when hospice personnel reminded me that the situation was technically terminal and I needed to discuss arrangements for her burial with her. It felt absolutely bizarre. The entire situation was incredulous.

We had lived in the same house for sixteen years. We often passed a small cemetery less than a quarter mile down the road. It occurred to me we had automatically assumed we would be buried there. However, in the moment, I also recalled when a cousin had taken us to my uncle's burial place in Pittsburgh. I was surprised to be entering a building. There was a waiting area that looked like a cozy inviting living room, complete with daily newspapers. We walked down a corridor of marble plaques. The mausoleum was open six days a week. The office for the cemetery personnel was there and arrangements could be made for mausoleum or in-ground burials. In fact we talked to someone and got an idea of what mausoleum burial crypts would cost. I liked it. It reminded me of the Church of Santa Croce in Florence where Dante, Petrarch and other famous Italians were buried. Nancy said she did not care for it. I thought it was dignified.

Here I was with Nancy in a hospital bed, in our TV room, facing death. I talked to her about mausoleums. She said she thought she preferred in-ground burial. Cremation was out of the question but she encouraged me to explore the mausoleum option. She was so tired, so exhausted. She said she had confidence in my decision, that I had good judgment.

I looked up "mausoleums" in the yellow pages and called several. I asked the pastor at our church about burial places. He was aware of one mausoleum in particular. Perhaps, because I was displeased by the fact most places were about a half-hour drive away from our home, the image of that little cemetery right down the road, kept popping into my head. However, I also wanted to explore mausoleums, as Nancy and I said we would be buried together and she wanted me to be comfortable with the decision as well. Inground burial did not appeal to me.

Accordingly, one lunch hour at work I drove to a cemetery and mausoleum which was just a few minutes down the road from my office. I had called ahead and the owner was expecting me. He showed me the mausoleum. I was shocked it was outside. I asked him if there was any heat in the winter or air conditioning in the summer. He said it was designed to be an outdoor mausoleum. He had heard of indoor mausoleums but he did not know of any in our area which were still selling crypts.

I tried to put that behind me and asked him which plots were available. He had several decent locations, including a double in the central area. We established a good rapport and basically I asked him to reserve the double. I would discuss it with Nancy and get back to him in a day or two. I was ready to leave when something caused me to ask about security. The mausoleum owner then escorted me to a vault which was at a desirable waist level and told me that some youths, bent on mischief, had recently broken the granite cover. It was really quite simple. It was about an inch thick. They just hit it with a hammer or a sledge hammer. Then they had pried through the metal cover and had pulled out the casket. He assured me they could not open the casket but that the youths did do some damage.

All of a sudden the ground was falling away under my feet. I found the open-air mausoleum to be totally unacceptable. Now I did not know what to do. My mind quickly ran to Nancy's preference for in-ground burial. The little cemetery down the road was suddenly the front runner. My knees buckled as I recalled hearing that it was completely sold out.

Back at work, I phoned the local church and they referred me to a specific local funeral home. I called the funeral home and spoke to the director. The first question was, "Did I belong to that church?" We had worshipped there for several years when we first moved into the area. Then we switched to an ethnic parish so Margaux could experience some of her cultural roots. Consequently, I was informed they could not sell me a burial plot unless the pastor approved it first.

My blood froze in my veins. I swallowed my pride and called him. I was surprised when I was put right through to him. I explained my circumstances and he said he would approve the transaction if there were any plots available. He was not sure, but he thought all the plots had been sold.

I hastily called the funeral director and we agreed to meet at the cemetery Saturday morning. Little did I know a week from that very Saturday, Nancy would be dead, her body would be in the funeral home and Margaux and I would be preparing for her funeral.

Margaux and I went to the cemetery that Saturday morning. Fortunately for us, it was a sunny day. The few available plots were at the back of the cemetery, near the railroad tracks. In our community, the railroad was the lifeblood of local history, the *raison d'etre* and a vestigial symbol of its uniqueness.

The railroad was not a problem for me, as I had very happy childhood memories which involved a New York commuter train. When I was about three or four years old, we lived in a second floor apartment. How well I remembered my glee each time I heard the oncoming train and ran to the window to look down and see it pass by on its way to the station.

The first plot he showed me was by a fence. It was so close to a huge old tree I could not comprehend how they could dig through the roots to open the grave. I was then shown a worn, tattered, oft-folded, hand-drawn map, which moved the plot a row or two to the center. The funeral director pointed at a huge pile of weeds and indicated something could be found in there. I didn't think so. He looked at the grimy map again and moved another row towards the center. He said he had a few plots at the end of the row. I carefully paced it out and was pleasantly surprised by the location. It was far enough away from the first tree, an equal distance from another, and not all that close to the railroad tracks.

I asked him if I could be buried there with her. He said this cemetery allowed only one body per grave. The cemetery in New York where my mother and father were buried allowed two deep. Here the bed rock was so thick they only allowed one. However, the good news was that the plot next to it was available, which I thought was great as I loved the trains. Nancy could have the plot nearer the road. I could have the one closer to the train tracks.

My guide then mentioned there was one more left at the end of the row, but that posed no problem because I immediately thought of Margaux. It was awkward and bizarre, but I then asked Margaux if she had thought about where she would want to be buried. She looked at me as if I had taken leave of my senses. I acknowledged that the question had come out of the blue, but that she should seriously consider this possibility, as the cemetery was virtually sold out. She would probably get married and want to be buried with her husband. However, as there was no way to predict how her life would progress, I wanted to buy the last plot just as insurance. It could always be sold or given to someone in need.

That day, decisions were made thinking only of the dead, and not of the living; I was not thinking about where new life could lead and how many other people could be involved in my future. Based on my life expectancy, I could conceivably live for another thirty years. As a dear friend later pointed out, my new life could take me anywhere, even overseas. Would I want to have my body returned here to be buried? This was not a question that could be answered permanently at that time. I was making decisions without taking any of this into consideration. I now realize that working in the moment, I had made plans as if my life had come to as final a conclusion as Nancy's.

I walked home from the cemetery and told Nancy all about our good fortune. She seemed happy and relieved that everything had been taken care of. She knew nothing about all the starts and stops I had encountered. There was no way for me to know she would never see her final resting place. There was no time. She was too weak. Invisibly, the cancer had penetrated too many parts of her poor body.

Miraculously, the next week, in response to my calls alerting them that Nancy did not have long to live, numerous family members and dear friends came to visit. At that moment, it was as if I had a sixth sense that the end was near. However, deep down, I still believed that she would pull it off one more time. 'The doctors had been wrong before, they will be wrong this time. Nancy is such a great fighter, she will make another comeback.' Perhaps because I was so emotionally involved in supporting her, most of the time I could not see the forest for the trees.

After the fact, however, it seemed everyone could see it clearly except for me. For example, several weeks after she died, several local merchants recollected their impressions of the last time she was in their shops. A green grocer reminisced, "I knew she did not have long to live the last time I saw her."

Her friend from her New York past, Harriet, came from a great distance. Sensing Nancy's weakness and exhaustion, it became a two-way day trip for her, rather than an overnight visit. As Harriet and Nancy said their good-byes, a sense of finality hung in the air that was so thick it was as if a blanket were smothering everything. The two of them wept when they took their leave. It was overwhelming for me to witness such an emotional moment.

Twenty-four hour nurses' aide care, an expensive luxury, also had significant drawbacks and disadvantages. Our home was no longer our own. Day and night, all doors were wide open to accommodate the stream of nurses' aides, nurses and hospice workers. The nursing service provided superb coverage: one person could not leave until the next arrived. However, I was unprepared for nocturnal shift changes. There was no private time for me to recoup. There was always someone in the house asking for this or that.

Weekdays, Nancy insisted I continue work at my new job. When I came home, Margaux would go off to her summer evening job and I was constantly wracked by tension. When I was out of the room, or away from Nancy, I longed to be with her. Each time I entered the room and saw her immobilized in the hospital bed, it tore me apart. I lived on this emotional see-saw for the last two weeks of her life.

Under the stress and strain of the situation, I was unaware that Margaux was struggling with her own overwhelming burden of being there for Nancy during the day without her father. I assumed she was okay with a chain of health care professionals going in and out. Many months later I would learn she was not okay. She had experienced the same ambivalent feelings I encountered. On top of that, she was not prepared to handle all the situations and decisions which arose.

Watching a loved one slowly die in front of your eyes, in your home, is an ordeal I cannot find words to describe. It feels akin to holding something precious in your cupped hands. It's right there. You have it. Then it starts to disintegrate. There's this powerful sinking feeling in the pit of your stomach as it slips between your straining fingers. I felt so helpless. The agony was excruciating when I realized I could not prevent it, no matter how hard I struggled, no matter how diligently and intently I tried.

During these last two weeks, there were times when Nancy's body was in the hospital bed, but she was not there. For example, one evening, Margaux and I went to a concert. When we came home, we rushed in to see Nancy. We felt death in the room. Looking at her, we thought she had died. Then, as if waking from a deep sleep, Nancy snapped out of it and came back to life.

I remembercd my grandmother telling me as a child that the dying received comfort when loved ones lit a blessed candle and prayed at their bedside. Accordingly, each night I lit a special candle, entered Nancy's room, and asked the aide for privacy so Nancy and I could pray together. When Margaux was not working, the three of us prayed. The candle was one that Nancy and I had purchased in Padua, Italy, at St. Anthony's shrine. We had never before had occasion to use it.

The evening of the Wednesday before she died, I was at Nancy's side, holding her hand as she lay in the hospital bed. I was talking softly to her but she was not responding. After a long while I became impatient and frustrated. In a louder voice, I called out to her as if to awaken her from her sleep, "Nancy, where are you?" "With the angels," she replied. Quickly and somewhat louder I asked, "But where are you?" She muttered something which was totally incomprehensible. "Tell me where you are. What do the angels look like?" I questioned. She turned her head to the side and seemed to go back to sleep.

Late that night I tried to find quiet time for myself. I sat in the darkened living room just outside her door. I lit a votive candle in front of an old statue of the Virgin Mary. I sat slumped and contemplative in my chair. Looking up, I stared at the shadow the candle and statue cast upon the wall. I saw the outline of an angel standing guard at Nancy's door. The angel was facing the doorway, with large powerful wings stretched back. When Margaux came home from work, I asked her to look at the shadow on the wall and tell me what she saw. She said she saw a shadow. I described what I saw. She did not. To me, it was as clear as could be.

Early the morning of the day Nancy died, I helped the nurses' aide turn her in the hospital bed. There was no noticeable response to her being moved. Her eyes did not open. She said nothing. I left for work knowing the hospice nurse would visit that morning. I was hopeful she would make it through the weekend, as not being with her always weighed heavily on my mind.

The hospice nurse called about 10:30 a.m. and informed me that Nancy had had pain and they had given her more morphine. Later that morning, Margaux called and told me the nurses' aide was acting strangely. Her mom was not moving and she had often stopped breathing and then resumed again, only after what seemed like an eternity. Around noon time, Margaux called me at work again, saying, "The nurse's-aide said mom has not been breathing for a few minutes." In disbelief, I said "What?"

Then the nurses' aide came on the extension and said, "Nancy has not breathed for over six minutes."

Margaux started to cry and scream in anguish. I hollered in the phone that I was on the way.

I drove in denial and disbelief, thinking how this nurses' aide seemed less skilled than some of the others. What does she know? Nancy will be alive when I get there. It must be a misunderstanding. The hospice nurse had said nothing about Nancy's death being imminent when she was there that morning, injecting the morphine.

When I got home, Margaux was in the driveway, crying. She ran to me, and I knew. Together we went into Nancy's room. Nancy's head was turned back and slightly towards the wall; her mouth was open, her eyes were closed, and her tongue was visible but not moving. All along she had turned her head towards the window, towards the light. There was no mistaking she was dead. I touched her hand and it was still warm.

What did I feel? For the most part, nothing. I felt numb. I felt only momentary relief it was all over, that she was not suffering. I felt turbulent emotions. Most importantly, I felt the need to hug Margaux and talk to her about what she was feeling.

Nancy died at approximately 11:30 on that Friday morning. After the funeral director and our friends left, Margaux and I stood on our patio. It was late afternoon. The day was mild, still and quiet. As we looked toward the west, in the direction of the setting sun, we were captivated by the sun, sky and clouds, interacting into clear soft shades of light blue and pink. We had the feeling Nancy was flying free and easy in the sky, in Heaven with the angels, looking down on us, happy and smiling. We felt terrible and in shock, but surely she was enjoying the reward she so justly deserved.

The next day I wrote this poem to Nancy. It expressed my feelings at that exact moment. As I sat at the computer composing, an uninterrupted stream of tears kept flowing from my eyes.

Mystical moments: birth and death.
And the myriad moments: the living in between.

Memories of meeting, loving—
Margaux being born.
Italy, France and 'Air Chance.'
Happy or sad, tender or tough
It all brought us closer together.

Why am I crying?
I know better.

We had fun.
Your illness only deepened our love.

After so many happy loving years,
(Yet so few!!!)
God called you to your well-earned reward.
Lord, Thy will be done.
I am joyous for you, yet I struggle with myself...
It is so hard to give you up,
Even for a little while.

Blessed with guardian angels on earth
Heavenly angels took you up to Him.

Rejoice with me!
I know you are happy there.
Busy, active and vital; helping out.
For surely Heaven can always use
Someone as beautiful and precious as you.
With Laura and Beatrice
You will continue your work
Inspiring all of us who remain.

Why do I grieve?
I know where you are. No doubt.
"Are you looking at those angels again?"
"Yes" was your last word to me.

I glimpsed celestial peace in your face.
You are in Heaven and in my heart,
Ever, forever, for eternity.

Time will fly
And so will I!
We will be together again.

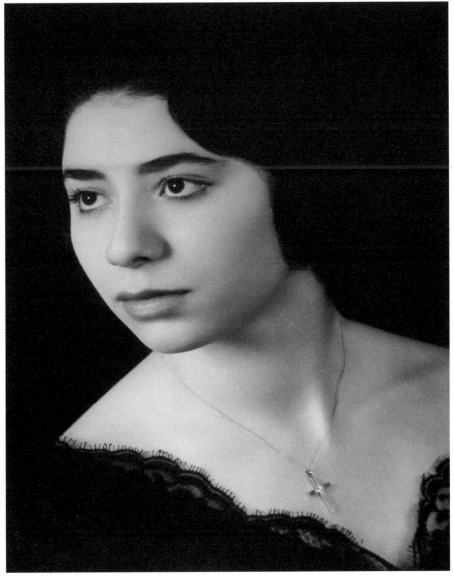

Nancy Spada Garbowski

Story of the Statue

After years of travel throughout Europe and countless hours spent in many museums, one of my dreams has been to own a hand-carved marble statue.

Several years ago, Nancy and I went to a major antique show in Atlantic City with our long time friends Julie and Jack.

Shortly after we ventured into the cavernous interior of the Convention Center, we discovered we had very different areas of interest. We therefore negotiated an arrangement to go off in pairs and meet at the main entrance every other hour.

The quantity and quality of the offerings was immense. Jack and I worked our way row by row, stopping now and then to examine something that appealed to either one of us. There was a stage at the back of the arena where the dealers appeared to be offering the highest quality merchandise. Jack admired a huge, elaborate wrought iron fence priced at several thousands of dollars. I admired expensive oil paintings and, in the back recesses of the stage area, I discovered a statue of a young woman surrounded by sheep.

The statue was striking in its intricacy, delicacy, charm and beauty. Regretfully, it had been through difficult times; the heads of all but one sheep had been broken off. Jack noticed the brim of the girl's hat was also broken. I observed her face was intact and she had a lovely expression. After having seen so many fragments and torsos in Europe, I was undaunted. A saleslady approached and started a conversation. I could not make a decision without my wife seeing the piece first. Happily, the statue was priced at just four hundred dollars. Jack and I returned to the main entrance every even hour that afternoon. Each time we returned, the ladies were no where to be seen. All the new treasures and delights we experienced now served but one purpose: to remind me I could not get that statue out of my mind. I decided to go back for a second look. No sooner did I walk up to the statue when the salesperson hurried over. "Yes, I was interested but I explained I could not find my wife and she would have to see it." The lady said she would sell the statue to me for half-price. I now found the situation maddening and irresistible. Sadly, I was unable to complete the transaction without Nancy's seeing it and the dealer was unable to hold it for me.

As we walked around, I paid no attention to the displays. I was looking for Nancy and Julie. Finally, at almost seven o'clock, we spied them several rows away. We asked where they had been, and our wives explained they had forgotten to meet us at the main entrance and were disappointed that everything was so very expensive. When I indicated I had found a statue, a treasure and a bargain, Nancy was adamantly opposed. However, after much cajoling, she agreed to go and only look at it.

After Nancy took one look at the statue, she immediately said, "No way!" Just then the saleslady came rushing up and informed me she had made a mistake. She should not have offered me the statue at half price, as that was what it had cost them. However, it was her mistake and she would honor that price for the rest of the day. The show closed in about an hour and a half, so I asked to talk privately with Nancy. Once again, Nancy was adamant there was no way I could bring that statue in our house. When I kept pressing her for a reason, she finally claimed it was so heavy it would break through the floor and fall into the basement.

Then Jack and Julie came over. Jack was an executive in a company involved in the construction and remodeling of homes. He assured Nancy the weight of the statue would not represent a problem. Logic and reason aside, Nancy still did not want the statue in our house.

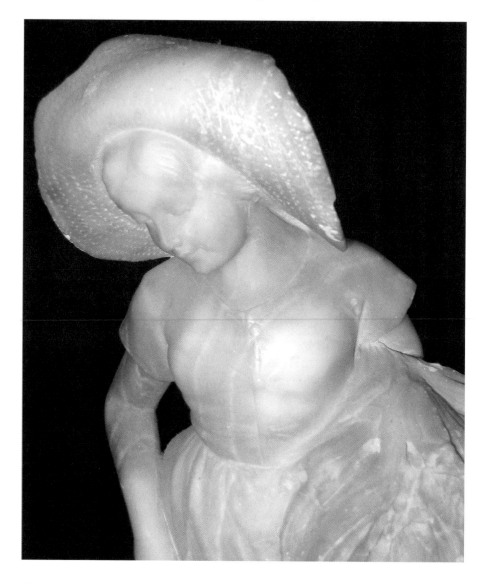

The statue was striking in its intricacy, delicacy, charm and beauty. Regretfully, it had been through difficult times; the heads of all but one sheep had been broken off. Jack noticed the brim of the girl's hat was also broken. I observed her face was intact and she had a lovely expression.

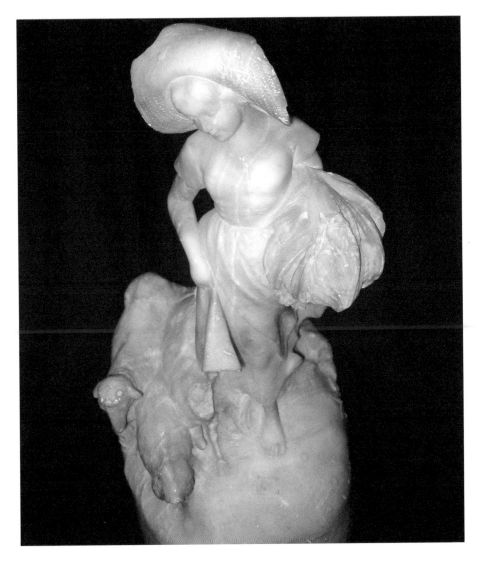

Multilated and mistreated, the statue exudes grace, beauty and style, illustrating that something broken and less than whole can possess an inner spirit and still be a work of art.

I came to possess this lovely statue through stress, conflict and turbulence. This characterized our relationship the last few years. Yet, we also managed to have fun and enjoy life. This statue is a symbol of our special relationship.

We all agreed to go to the bathrooms before heading over to the casino. I just could not get the statue out of my mind. As soon as Nancy came out of the washroom, I told her I had to have the statue. Surprisingly, she stopped her opposition.

I hurried back to the dealer and told the salesperson to wrap it up. When I presented my charge card I was told they could only accept cash or a personal check. Julie immediately offered to write a personal check to the dealer and said that I could pay her back the next day.

It was another adventure carrying the fifty pound statue to the parking garage. Jack helped me by taking turns. Eventually, we got it safely to the car.

At midnight, Jack graciously helped me set the statue on the floor of our dining room. I selected the dining room as it had a solid concrete floor so Nancy could sleep that night without worrying about our hardwood floor's sustaining the weight. I wrote Julie a check for the amount and expressed my heartfelt thanks to both of them. I could not have done it alone.

When I woke up the next morning, Nancy was not in bed next to me. I wandered through the house looking for her and finally found her in the dining room, on her knees, staring at the statue. She was so engrossed that at first she did not even notice my presence. Then she turned and said, "This girl has the sweetest expression on her face. The rocks and sheep are the way I imagine Alfadena to be." Alfadena was a tiny mountain village in the Abruzzi region of Italy, the birthplace of Nancy's grandparents.

From that moment on we both loved the statue and we were later fortunate enough to be able to visit Alfadena together. The sights we experienced and the people we met reinforced Nancy's connection to the statue. The shepherd girl from Alfadena is a fitting symbol of this book. Mutilated and mistreated, the statue exudes grace, beauty and style, illustrating that something broken and less than whole can possess an inner spirit and still be a work of art.

100

I came to possess this lovely statue through stress, conflict and turbulence. This characterized our relationship the last few years. Yet, we also managed to have fun and enjoy life. This statue is a symbol of our special relationship.

Now, here's what you can do.....

* Try your best to monitor, observe and most importantly, support your loved one in general. Whereas Nancy sensed when to fight and when to stop fighting, not all patients understand the distinction. I have heard of individuals diagnosed with cancer who were dead and buried in months. Frightened by the diagnosis, they gave up the fight. Others resist death, bedridden for months and months, fighting with every last ounce of energy, every last breath.
* Try not to be selfish, expecting your loved one to endure all the treatments just to be there for you.
* Discuss insomnia with your physician if it becomes a serious problem for you or other family members.
* Remember, it is often better for all involved if the terminally ill can make their own final arrangements. This gives them a sense of control and peace of mind that everything will be consistent with their last wishes. This also takes a lot of pressure off the family.
* If an ill person is physically unable to visit the funeral home or go to the cemetery, the best you can do is to discuss as many of the details as possible and involve them in the decision-making process, while still being sensitive to observe just how much they can handle.
* The sooner you address these issues, the better and remember that friends, neighbors, and clergy can all provide critical input.
* Try not to be hard on yourself, the care provider, for being preoccupied with ever unending matters and thus

not being able to be at your loved one's bedside all the time.

* Men innately want to solve problems and cure ailments. However, if at a point of no return, where there is no chance of recovery, the biggest gift a male caregiver can give is to "go with the flow" (rather than try to solve), and to listen carefully to what their loved one wants and needs at that particular point in time.

* Oftentimes the terminally ill need to hear their loved ones say, "It's OK to let go," which helps them peacefully accept their impending death.

CHAPTER 7
Grieving

Jan Kochanowski is one of Poland's greatest poets and authors. Renowned for many works, his greatest legacy concerns the death of his beloved four year old daughter, Ursula. The great poet, shattered and heartbroken, poured his soul into the Laments. At one point in my grieving I read this very lengthy poem in its entirety. I annotated the following sections because they seemed particularly poignant and meaningful to me at the time.

> The void that fills my house is so immense....
> All your old haunts have turned to haunts of pain...
> [Lament 8]

> But is there any truth in what we're told
> About your power to purge our human thought
> Of all its dread, and raise up the distraught
> Spirit to heaven, to the highest sphere
> Where angels dwell beyond distress and fear?
> [Lament 9]

> ...where did you go?
> Is it a place or a country that we know?
> Wherever you may be—if you exist—
> Take pity on my grief. O presence missed,
> Comfort me, haunt me; you whom I have lost.
> Come back again, be shadow, dream or ghost.
> [Lament 10]

> I'll turn, if I'm not healed,
> to a marble pillar in a field,
> A monument to pain, a standing stone
> That weeps and bleeds like living flesh and bone.
> [Lament 15]

It was for her, my son, things turned out best,
So dry your tears. Believe. Take comfort. Rest.
You must accept, although your wound's still raw,
The rule and sway of universal law
And fill your heart with new peace, banish pain.
   [Lament 19]
   Laments by Jan Kochanowski.
   (Translated by Baranczak and Heaney)

A friend of mine once expressed amazement over the composure an individual demonstrated at the funeral of her husband. Having been through such grief myself, it was now clear that she was in such a deep profound state of shock that her body went into a protective state of numbness.

Likewise, in the film *Godfather III*, there is a scene where Al Pacino's daughter is shot dead on the steps of the Palermo opera house. Pacino ran to her and took her in his arms. His mouth opened to scream and no sound came out.

When I first experienced this scene, I felt it to be a trifle forced and stagey. I chalked it up to the director's, Francis Ford Coppola's, trying to be artistic. Now that I have experienced profound grieving, I look back on this scene and I marvel at its true-to-life artistry. There are times the pain is so deep and intense that it actually obliterates all feelings and all sensations. Michael Corleone's pain, stuck in his throat like a stray fishbone, is beyond expression.

In time, this natural sedation wears off and the pain blows in like a primitive, wild, uncontrollable fall hurricane, sweeping you off your feet, and crashing down all the walls and defenses with which you have surrounded yourself.

This analogy is important to help you understand the danger you are in. It's easy to see why older people sometimes die and get buried with their spouses. Others follow in just a few months. Some never date or remarry. Some grieve their loss for many years before resuming an active life and accepting someone new in their lives.

Loving and being loved is a gift from God. You can't make it happen. You can, however, open yourself up to it or you can shut yourself down to it. Unfortunately, the pain and numbness of grieving can cut you off from both giving and receiving love. It takes courage and conviction to push hard to regain strength and mobility and open yourself, once again, to love.

When a lost loved one casts a big shadow in your life, you may experience emptiness. I felt alone just as Nancy was alone in her final days. She too had family and friends there to support her. Yet, she had to turn to her inward strength and go to her inner space to come to peace with her impending death. She did not speak the last three days because she was too tired and she did not need to speak. Her work was internal and deeply personal and private. This, too, was how grieving felt to me.

You can't help but miss all the activities your loved one engaged in; all of the things you did together. You may even miss the "honey-do" lists. Honey, do this and honey do that.

Grieving is also an endless string of dark, grey, gloomy, drizzly days. Something deep inside your being longs for blue skies and sunlight but, imperceptibly, you adjust your lifestyle to the unending rain. You keep an umbrella by your door, and in your car.

Hopefully, grieving progresses through processing, confronting, accepting, acknowledging, and, eventually, to healing. However, this is not a clear-cut process. It's a little like driving through a long dark tunnel. No sooner do your eyes adjust to the darkness and the glaring beams surrounding you, when suddenly, you emerge into the bright sunlight and you're blinded for a few moments, as your eyes struggle to make another adjustment.

"Grief, like manure, is meaningless until we learn how to use it. We use manure to grow beautiful flowers or delicious food. Similarly, we need to make something good come from our grief. Making our grief meaningful can be the antidote to despair and suffering as well as the stepping-stone to personal growth and achievement. We can choose to turn great personal tragedy into life-affirming action or personal change. The more we reach toward life, instead of withdrawing into our tragedy, and the more we aim for achievement or accomplishment, the more we expand our own possibilities. To transform ourselves does not mean to become something we are not, but to expand ourselves to our farthest reaches, to achieve our greatest potential. It is from reaching beyond ourselves, beyond our sorrow, that we are transformed," wrote Judith Tatelbaum in her book *Courage to Grieve.*

This is the desired state, the goal and end result of successfully completing the grieving process. However, to get there requires we navigate a long, winding and arduous road.

Anger is also an integral part of grieving. When unprocessed, this anger can fester within you like cancer itself and infiltrate the rest of your life. Several weeks after Nancy died, I was reading Judy Tatelbaum's book on grieving. She emphasized the importance of surfacing unprocessed anger. I reflected upon this passage and decided I felt no anger. It wasn't Nancy's fault. She couldn't help having cancer.

However, over time, with deeper thought, I recognized several types of anger. I felt anger over Nancy's diminished companionship the last several years. For example, she had had to give up tennis and I had to find new partners. Whereas we had the time and money, her illness restricted our travel opportunities. I also resented the cancer attacking her mind and her not knowing me, nor knowing when I was helping her. Furthermore her tendency to say something that was under-cutting and corrosive to my self-esteem and then turn around to berate me for a lack of self-confidence, also greatly troubled me. Eventually, I also found it ironic that while idolizing Nancy, I had been oblivious to the fact that her needs were often accomplished at my emotional and physical expense. Most of all, over time, I recognized my overwhelming resentment over her dying and leaving me alone to take care of Margaux, with no family in the area.

About six weeks after Nancy died, I went to a three day, job-related, off-site culture change seminar. One exercise at this meeting involved our relaxing and listening to soft, soothing, music with our eyes closed, while the facilitator encouraged us to breathe slowly, and to count backwards from ten, one at a time, for each exhale. We were asked to visualize how we were at work, how we worked together. Then the facilitator told us it was the end of the day, to get in the car, pull into the driveway and visualize how you were for your family when you went home. Five years earlier, I would have thought about leaving problems at work, thus not being agitated or stressed when I came home. Now it was excruciatingly painful to realize there was no one to come home to, other than Nancy's presence in the colorful pale blue and bright pink hues in the sky. The pain was so intense, I almost left the room.

I have a history of sleepwalking when under extreme stress or duress. Back home, early that Sunday morning, I experienced an old nightmare, of being trapped in a strange place in the dark and not being able to find my way out. When I got up later in the morning, I had a mighty yawn and felt a muscle pull in my jaw. Getting ready for church, I had a massive sneeze and I felt a sharp pain in my lower back. This pain was to stay with me for days. Gradually, I started to realize that I was indeed very tense and upset.

When she first died, I envisioned Nancy in Heaven singing with the angels. Now, however, all I could see was her body in the casket. She always had beautiful skin and took meticulous care of her face with expensive creams, lotions and restoratives. Now all I envisioned was her dead body in the casket, the skin drying out, decaying, drawing tighter and tighter over her skull.

Something beautiful and positive had somehow changed into something sad, morbid and depressing. Since I was very connected to Nancy, I had always experienced what she was experiencing physically. For example, when she had nausea from chemotherapy, I, too, felt nauseous. Now that she was dead, I felt what it was like to be in her decaying body.

Looking back, in my sorrow, it seems to me the process of grieving is much like a beach. One night, during our last shared vacation in Cape May, New Jersey, the sun was setting behind the lighthouse and it caused the sea to glisten and shimmer with such intensity; it almost hurt my eyes. It was as if there were a huge swarming school of Cape May diamonds floating on the surface of the water, reflecting bright rays of light in every which way. It was high tide and each incoming wave lapped higher up on the beach than the last one had.

My pain was as full as that high tide. When an unexpectedly large wave crashed into me, I was knocked off my feet, my glasses fell off and I was disoriented. It felt as if my entire world were out of control. For a split second, I panicked and feared drowning. Then, the wave receded and I fought back against the force that had sucked me in. Next was a feeling of relief and the following waves were softer and gentler. I almost did not feel them. Luckily, I found my glasses. I was exhilarated, back in control of my destiny. I was now eager to live life to the fullest, just the way we used to, in spite of her illness. Then unexpectedly, another powerful wave pulled my feet out from under me and I was back in the surf, thrashing around, simultaneously swallowing and spitting up salty sea water.

When the tide turns, each incoming wave is imperceptibly shorter than the last, except for the occasional big one. Friends told me these hurtful waves would diminish in frequency. However, right after Nancy died, these waves seemed to be coming in hard and fast. I had to believe this cycle too would pass.

Within a month of Nancy's death I joined a widow and widowers' support group. Meeting after meeting we talked about healing, processing and moving forward. Even persons a year or two from their loss were stuck in their grief. They told me I had a long way to go. I refused to accept that notion.

Nancy had always processed her losses and moved forward, inspiring others. I knew that was what she would want me to do. "I am not going to be like the others, wallowing in my grief. I am going to face my feelings, accept them, process them and move on with my life. This is how Nancy would want me to behave. This is what I want to do."

It was almost three months to the day after Nancy died. I had attended an all-day seminar which ended earlier than expected. On the way home, I decided to go to the cemetery, even though the sun was setting and the late fall light was rapidly waning. It was a brisk kind of cold with a moderate wind. I felt the tears welling up as I turned into the cemetery. By the time I got to her grave, I was wailing, sobbing, and whining like a hurt animal. Suddenly I stopped, thinking that Nancy would not want me to carry on like this. In fact, she would tell me to "cut it out!" I never ever saw her carry on like this.

When I got home, I was delighted to discover a book order from a bank in Florida. I had not sold any books since Nancy died. I made a quick and easy meal, watched television and started preparing the book order for shipment. Being in the house, I could feel hurt, pain, loss and an antsy feeling I now regarded as an integral part of living.

I was in the kitchen with tape and scissors when out of nowhere, random, powerful thoughts came to mind. "I'm okay. Nancy's okay. Margaux's okay. We got through it together. Successfully. Nancy is free of pain. Margaux and I helped her make her peace with life here on earth. She's in a better place."

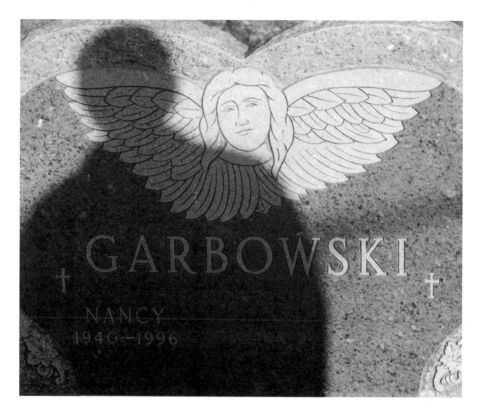

I felt the tears welling up as I turned into the cemetery. By the time I got to her grave, I was wailing, sobbing and whining like a hurt animal.

"I'm okay. I'm selling books again. I'm making a presentation to a business group tomorrow. Financially, all is well. I have this house."

"Margaux's okay. She's back at school. She has decided to go ahead with her winter semester of study in London."

It could have been much much worse. Nancy could have suffered a lot of pain. She did not. I could have been ruined financially. I was not. Cancer attacked all three of us with all its fury and together, we got through it.

"The first weekend I was alone I had a tight, crushing feeling in the pit of my stomach. I could have died from an anxiety attack. I got through that. I've felt the depth and fullness of my grief and—I'm okay."

A feeling of calm and peace came over me, momentarily reminding me of the peace Nancy enjoyed on the threshold of leaving this life for the next. It felt wonderfully affirming, not only of life, but of the total process which is both life and death. Now, there was nothing to fear. Nothing to be anxious about. The worst that could happen to me was that I would die. Nancy died under extremely adverse and trying circumstances. She did it with dignity and grace. We did that together. Hopefully, I too can do it when the time comes, even if I'm alone.

Less than two months after Nancy died, Margaux expressed similar deep feelings. "What I feel from mom isn't something I can rationally explain. I just feel her. There's a warmth in my chest and that keeps me strong. It is God's love. But now there is more warmth, and that is mom. It is hard to describe, but I feel them both with me all of the time. Just like God is not physically there, still, I know, He is there. I was talking to a friend who came to the funeral. She believes life on earth is our purgatory or hell, and when we die we go right to heaven. That seems as though it could be possible because of the way I saw mom go. She suffered and had pain throughout her life but, when it was time to die, she was with the angels, going straight up."

Another aspect of grieving for both Margaux and me was processing the fact that we were not in the room with Nancy when she died. In time, Margaux and I were able to talk about how we felt. Nancy insisted I go off to work each day, no questions asked. However, it was even more difficult for Margaux as she had been in the house when her mother died. I kept reassuring her it was not her fault. There was no way for her to know. There had been a lot of confusion that day.

During this discussion, one thing led to another and I remembered a visiting priest conducting a parish mission just the year before. Nancy insisted on going every night. It was Wednesday. Father had finished his prepared remarks and was entertaining questions from the congregation. I do not recall the question which produced the following unforgettable answer.

"Several years ago, my mother was in the hospital. She was dying. I had stayed with her night and day. One night a nurse came in and told me I needed to go home and get some sleep. I thanked her for her concern but I firmly told her to leave me with my mother.

A few hours later this nurse came back into the room. She remarked at how drawn I looked and how much I needed to rest to maintain my health. I told her I just wanted to be there with my mother.

She came back a third time and assured me that my mother was doing just fine. She was stable, nothing would happen and they would call me right away if there was any turn for the worse. It was already past midnight. She told me to go and get just a few hours of sleep...to come back in the morning...that everything would be okay.

Well, I listened to her and went home and fell asleep. The phone rang at six a.m. It was the hospital calling to tell me my mother had died.

I hurried back to her room. When I entered she was still warm. I closed the door and I wept. I prayed to God. 'God, you gave me a special calling to be a priest. I have been with thousands of dying people. Why, oh, why, did you not let me be with my mother when she died? This is my calling, my mission!'

A nurse came to the door to see how I was since I had been in the room alone with the body for a long time. I told her to leave.

I kept asking God, 'Why did she die without me? Why did she die alone? How could you let me minister to so many strangers and not comfort my mother during her last moments?'

Another nurse came to the door. I was in such a state of agitation I told her to go away.

I prayed and prayed to God, not understanding how something like this could happen. Finally God said to me, 'Mario, do not be upset. I did not need you to be here last night as I was with your mother.' "

CHAPTER 8
Their Spirit Lives On

"Gramps loved mallards," Lorna, recalls. "On the one year anniversary of his death, my daughter, Michelle, and I were drawn to a nearby cemetery by a flock of Canadian geese. While watching them on a frozen pond, we suddenly noticed a single mallard. Every year thereafter I would go to that cemetery on the anniversary of his death. Every year I would observe a flock of geese, and a solitary mallard. One year I could not contain my curiosity. I went to the cemetery the day before the anniversary of his death. Sure enough, there was a flock of geese, but no mallard. The next day the mallard was there to greet me and my daughter, but, the day after the anniversary, the mallard had disappeared. That mallard symbolized Gramps' spirit, his soul. It was so comforting to think that he would be with us in such a special way, especially when mourning his death was still so difficult."

Nancy died on Friday. That weekend, we worked on her funeral arrangements. The night before Nancy's viewing at the funeral home, Margaux and I decided to make a tape of Nancy's favorite music. This collection consisted of opera, classical music and Broadway show tunes. Huddled in front of the stereo system which Margaux had bought us for a 25th wedding anniversary gift, we compiled joyous, upbeat music. Suddenly, I felt Nancy's presence in the room, right there in front of me. I could see nothing, hear nothing, smell nothing. But I could feel her right there. I asked Margaux if she felt anything. She said, "No." Then the presence dissipated. It felt as if Nancy was looking over us at work, approving of the selections. Later that evening I felt her again. This time, determined to seize the moment, I reached out to put my arms around her. Instantly Nancy was gone.

Then again, the night Nancy was laid out at the funeral home, after all the visitors had left, Margaux said she wanted to take a picture of her mother in the casket. She asked me if that was weird. I said "No." I had a photograph of a great-grandfather of mine in the casket at the edge of the open grave in the cemetery. I explained that cultures vary, that some folks do not take photos of the deceased while others do. However, I also reminded her that her mother did not approve of the practice.

Margaux insisted on going home to get a camera. I remembered she had been having problems with her equipment so I offered her mine. In a few minutes she came back with her camera and she took one or two photos of Nancy in the open casket.

When the pictures were developed, all I heard was a tearful, emotional, "The pictures did not come out. I hate this camera."

Almost a year later, Margaux was sorting out some school photos for her book when she casually showed me a picture and asked me what I thought it was.

It looked like one of those time release photos where automobile lights appear as lines. The picture was very fuzzy and faded, but there were two jagged circular lines.

"That's the picture of mom in the casket," Margaux stated.

In disbelief I blurted out, "You told me nothing turned out."

"Well, this is how it came out," she replied.

With her explanation, I could now make out the blurry outline of the casket. The jagged circular lines were the floor lamps on either side of the casket. When I looked closely and carefully, I could barely make out her head but then remembered that she had been laid-out with her head to the right. In the photo it was a darker fuzzy ball.

My conclusion was Nancy did not want her picture taken and a force from beyond the grave had reached out to distort the picture beyond any reasonable recognition. Several years later, thanks to being introduced to Tai-chi, I would look at this photograph as capturing Nancy's energy field and her actual vital life force,

115

hovering around her loved ones, who had gathered to pay their last, loving respects.

Several days after the funeral, I needed something from the attic. Having climbed the steep stairs, I turned on the light and was bewildered by the sight of a broken picture frame dangling from a rafter. The glass was lying unbroken on the rough wooden floor and the contents of the frame, Nancy's mother's photo, lay curled, but not damaged, on the floor. Even the dead seemed to be reaching out to make contact with Nancy. An eerie sensation passed through me.

About three months after Nancy died, I forced myself to be alone in our house for the weekend. At one point I thought I could smell her. I went from room to room. Living room, no smell. Bathroom, yes, I could smell her presence. Hallway, less smell. TV room, no smell. Back to the bathroom. Yes, she was still with me.

I remembered previously reaching out and driving her away. Consequently, this time I stood there quietly, enjoying her presence. It felt good to have some contact, any contact. I yearned to hug her, kiss her, above all to speak with her just one last time. But this could never be. Quietly, I closed my eyes, did not move, and enjoyed what I could. It was as if she were telling me all was well.

Margaux, too, had her own personal encounter with Nancy's spirit when she was back-packing in Brussels with two young women, just six months after her mother's death. They had arrived in a strange city after dark, with no map and no idea where the youth hostel was situated. The streets were deserted. As midnight approached, her two companions started to panic. Fearful for their safety, they just wanted to go back home.

Sure enough, Margaux felt her mother's presence, guiding her. She was supremely confident that no harm would befall her. She was sure her mother would lead her to the hostel. By 1:00 a.m. Margaux and her two friends had safely checked in. Although she would never do any-thing like that again, the experience did allow her to feel the vitality of her mother's protective, loving spirit.

Nine months later, a local breast cancer support group, Living Beyond Breast Cancer, dedicated their annual meeting to a 'celebration of Nancy's life.' The morning of the conference, after wrestling with the decision of what to wear, I finally chose and put on a nice designer shirt. While knotting the tie, I once again had a powerful inexplicable feeling which caused me to remove both the shirt and tie and put them back on the hanger. I then reached up, and took down a department store bag, which contained a shirt Nancy had personally chosen for me just two months before her death. I knew it was there, but I could not bring myself to wear it and the beautiful matching tie. At this exact moment, I felt Nancy's presence in the room, saying in her inimitable way, "What are you saving that shirt for? It's going to rot in that bag before you wear it! This conference is important. Put on that new shirt and tie right now."

The tears rolled down my face as I removed all the packing pins and new-shirt stuffing. The tears continued as I cut off the price tags. I was happy to be wearing the new combination. I could feel her right there with me. Such visits were so rare, yet so special. These were tears of both unbridled joy and bottomless sorrow and sadness.

Even Margaux, while shopping for a new automobile, several months later, felt strongly influenced by Nancy. Her mother had expressed a strong desire to give her a car upon graduation. Now, however, it seemed appropriate to give Margaux this gift in advance, during her Senior year. After narrowing the search down to a previously owned BMW, a VW Jetta or a sporty type car, Margaux's heart was set on the BMW. However, the BMW had 75,000 miles on it and I believed a new car was preferable to a used one.

Just before we were ready to go and look at the sports car one more time, the phone rang. It was the salesperson calling to discuss various options. Margaux answered the phone in the kitchen. Meanwhile, in the living room, I felt Nancy's presence entering the room and sitting on the sofa opposite me. I could almost hear her voice, "You shimaneeds, get going. Margaux needs a new car. She loves that sporty car. It won the JD Power award and it also earned a Consumers Report recommendation. I don't know what's holding you back. Get going. That's the car for her." Nancy always had a sense of what was hot. I started sobbing uncontrollably. Once again, I felt so very close to her.

Margaux heard a commotion and after hanging up, rushed into the living room and asked what was going on. We then talked and Margaux, too, shared her intuitions. Her Godfather had worked in the automotive business and he had always dreamed of owning a Trans Am. Therefore, when he died in a plane crash, his widow had the likeness of the car etched into his monument. Nancy had died the same day of the year that he died. Margaux explained to me that these two signs felt significant to her. Consequently, we signed on the line for the sporty car that very evening.

Several years after this occurrence, Margaux became engaged to Jason and I was invited to visit them in Virginia to look at wedding dresses. While loading my car on a beautiful summer morning, two white butterflies fluttered towards me, circled my body and then disappeared across the lawn. Shortly thereafter, while closing down the house, I happened to look out the window and noticed several large groups of white butterflies. Their presence was bright white against the dark green summer vegetation. Drawn outside, I discovered butterflies everywhere. I then recalled that Nancy had been fascinated by butterflies the last summer of her life.

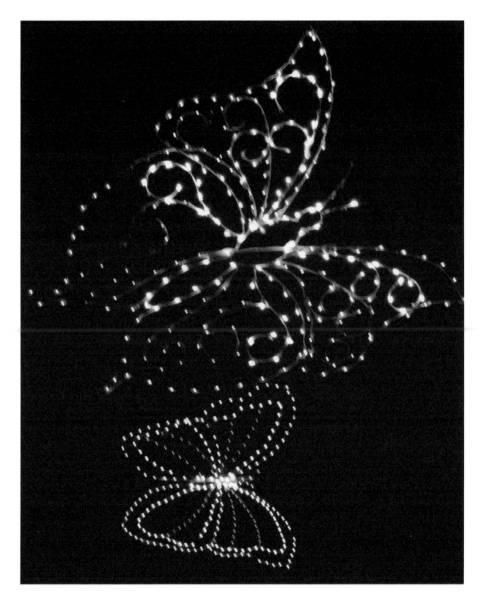

For months after this visit to Margaux and Jason's, pairs of butterflies constantly pierced my consciousness at home, on local roads and on the highways . . . In each pair of butterflies I felt the presence of both Nancy and my friend Lorna, constantly reminding me that although I was a single parent facing the daunting prospect of my "little girl's" getting married, I was not alone.

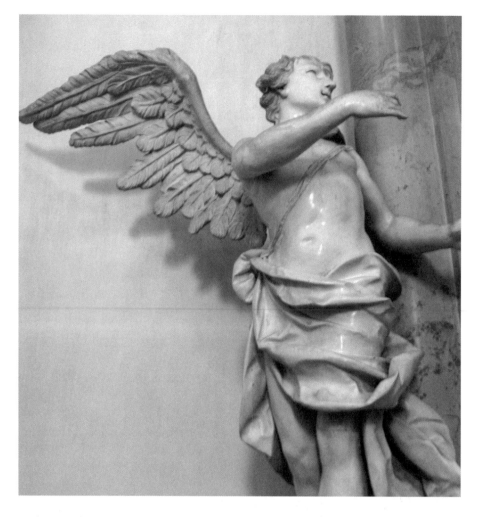

Looking over my shoulder, my eye was drawn to a marble statue of a winged angel to the left of a modest altar. The shape of the extended wing and the angelic face, turned to the right, stirred memories and transported me back in time to the night when just such an angel stood guard at the door to Nancy's room where she lay on her deathbed.

For months after this visit to Margaux and Jason's, pairs of butterflies constantly pierced my consciousness at home, on local roads and on the highway. Even when out of state this phenomenon occurred over and over again. In each pair of butterflies I felt the presence of both Nancy and my friend Lorna, constantly reminding me that although I was a single parent facing the daunting prospect of my "little girl's" getting married, I was not alone.

The wonderful, exhilarating sensation of Nancy's being close to me in spirit occurred in a Benedictine Abbey in Amorbach, Germany. While touring the legendary open-aired Christmas markets in Bavaria with a college alumni group, we were honored with an organ recital. The Church was not heated and the damp cold penetrated to the bone. A group of grammar school children sang Christmas carols for us and their enthusiasm warmed the soul. Then the magnificent organ concert began. Looking over my shoulder my eye was drawn to a marble statue of a winged angel to the left of a modest side altar. The shape of the extended wing and the angelic face, turned to the right, stirred memories and transported me back in time to the night when just such an angel stood guard at the door to Nancy's room where she lay on her deathbed. As I fixed my gaze on this heavenly figure I actually felt Nancy sitting right there next to me, enjoying the organ concert with me. The feeling was so intense, so powerful, so loving and so positive, that it caused tears of joy and happiness to stream down my face for the entire half hour.

There is no doubt in my mind: their spirit lives on!

Now here's what you can do.....

* Be open-minded when it comes to the possibility of comforting spiritual experiences.
* When you sense it is appropriate, don't be afraid to share some of your spiritual experiences. For example, while hosting a widow and widowers' discussion of an opera, a comment was made about spirituality. This, in turn, led to virtually every individual sharing some personal spiritual experience with the group. It was a most moving and comforting experience for all.

CHAPTER 9
Life Goes On

Recalling the famous line from *Richard III*, "All is at sixes and sevens," after Nancy's death, nature seemed turned inside out and in turmoil. As I was living alone for the first time in my life, the house was very quiet and it often felt like time was standing still. To appreciate the ying and yang of my situation, envision a stately swan, gliding along a tranquil lake. However, beneath this calm tableau, the webbed feet of the swan are paddling furiously, just out of sight.

Over and over again, I felt my loss, at many times and in many places. For example, each time I visited Nancy at the cemetery, even before I got out of the car, I felt very emotional. I remember one time in particular when I found, at her grave, a bouquet of carnations and mixed flowers which had been left earlier that day by Margaux and her friend. Wrapped in a colorful plastic, it was lying on its side on the ground. I wept bitterly at the sight. The bouquet symbolized my pain, hurt and loss. Nancy could not reach out and hold the bouquet. She could not smell the fragrant carnations. She could not see its colorful beauty on this bleak cold overcast wintry day. The bouquet just lay there on its side, helpless and alone.

Intense grieving can occur at virtually any moment. Five months after Nancy's death, Margaux embarked on a semester in London. I agreed to visit her during spring break. I saw this as an opportunity for us to talk and process feelings. Together, we decided to take a week's vacation in Florence, Italy. While there, Margaux and I walked by the Bonciani Hotel where the three of us had stayed in 1985. Predictably, the experience made Margaux and I sad and stirred bitter-sweet emotions.

Planning our vacation, I decided to combine something new with something familiar by selecting

Siena. Once in Florence, Margaux and I made inquiries, then went to the bus station and carefully mapped out our trip. The morning of the transfer, everything went smoothly. We arrived at the terminal, purchased our tickets and, with precision, boarded the bus. We were happy to be going on this extra excursion. While waiting for the bus to pull out, I started reading about Siena in my old travel guide book. As I leafed through the pages, I suddenly came across a Siena section with the following pen notations in Nancy's handwriting: "Sita bus line near train station. Florence to Siena by bus - 1 1/2 hours." It felt as if a bullet had torn through my heart. Uncontrollable tears poured down my face. One moment I felt warm and good. It was as if Nancy were right there, sitting next to us on the bus, just like the good old days. Then I felt a terrible, overwhelming sadness because Nancy wanted to take this trip, she wanted to see Siena and she never would. The finality of her death ripped through me. Once again, life felt so fragile, so fleeting.

Other forms of grieving can also occur with alarming regularity. Initially, Margaux had nightmares every month on the exact day of her mother's death. In one dream, she was sleeping with her mother to keep her comfortable as her mother was not well. Nancy was having trouble breathing. She woke Margaux up, asked her to help, and died in Margaux's arms.

During another nightmare, Margaux's mother had skin cancer with lesions and she started tearing at the skin, ripping off the cancerous tissue. "I yelled at her to stop or she would really hurt herself. Her eyes were all buggy and she would not listen to me. She just kept tearing away at her skin."

Gradually, Margaux's dreams started to abate in intensity. On one occasion, she experienced a dream within a dream. Margaux was with a friend. The two took a nap. In her sleep her mother came to her and said, "I still love you." Margaux said it was exciting to hear her voice again. When mother and daughter took a little walk, Margaux could feel her mom's hand on her

124

back. She woke up next to her friend and emerged from the dream, within the dream, to find herself in her familiar room. Alone. For Margaux, the overall effect of this particular dream was good and positive.

In time, Margaux would confide in me, "If you just open yourself up, I can feel her sometimes. It's not the same as when she was alive, but I can definitely feel her."

We take many things for granted when we have them. For example, think of the expensive ring on your finger. If it's a wedding band, the selection and the ritual during which it was slipped on your finger were exhilarating peaks in your life. Then, over the years, you almost forget that you are wearing it. Likewise, Margaux grieved long and hard over never hearing her mother's voice again. Never hearing her yell at her for some minor transgression such as throwing clothes on the floor in her room. Never holding her hand again.

Similarly, a loved one often experiences almost debilitating bouts of insomnia, not knowing how to sleep without a partner. I found it difficult. It takes a long time to get accustomed to the cold empty bed and the loss of Nancy's gentle touch, her hug, her caress.

When the first spring arrived, Nancy was not here to see it for the first time in over fifty years. The first Palm Sunday without Nancy was also particularly bad. I recalled her love for weaving palms into elaborate decorative pieces to decorate the Church altar on Palm Sunday. Then we always brought her masterpieces home to celebrate the Holiday.

Likewise on Nancy's first absentee birthday, life felt like a tease. For years we had worked so hard to create a meaningful relationship. Once I'd tasted it, it was cruel to have it taken away. Crueler still was the fact that I was constantly surrounded by all the articles Nancy had so lovingly collected and cherished, whereas, in death, she took nothing with her.

The process of selecting and designing a memorial marker proved to be still another significant factor in Margaux's and my grieving process. I chose to work with a retired talkative gentleman, Frank, who ran his business from his house. A very perceptive fellow, he clearly enjoyed working with people and offered a wealth of experience. He was especially keen about working with Margaux and me as we were designing a stone based upon a drawing by Margaux. After Frank showed us photos of several other individual gravestones he had helped design and execute, I was sure he was our man.

Margaux and I selected a Missouri red granite stone four feet in length and just as tall. Where the outline of the stone simulated the wings of an angel, Margaux drew a unique, yet simple shape; an angel's face turned to the side. When the drawings came back from Vermont, the face had been modified, yet it retained the sense of Margaux's drawing. Grape vines were also sketched along both sides near the bottom of the stone, representing one of my passions.

While we were working on revisions to the drawings, a turbulent moment in Margaux's grieving occurred. The drawing had the family name in the center in large characters. To one side was Nancy's name, the year of her birth and the year of her death. To the other side was my first name. At one point Margaux insisted my year of birth be engraved. I indicated I was not comfortable with that. It felt as if I were just waiting to die, to complete the design.

In a subsequent revision I was uncomfortable with even my name being there. I didn't know how to tell Margaux. At one point I said, "I don't want my name on the stone."

Margaux challenged me right back, "Why not?"

Remembering my previous conversation with a friend concerning death and burial, I responded, "I don't know when I'll die. I don't know what my life holds in store for me."

Margaux was instantly upset. She broke into tears saying, "Well fine, put my name there. I can't bear the thought of mom buried there forever all by herself. No one with her."

"That's not what I meant to say. I'm simply saying I don't want my name on there right now." I realized I had confused Margaux; yet, the intensity of her response took me by surprise.

When we met with Frank and discussed removing the name, Margaux stormed out of the office to sit in the car, crying. Frank asked me what was the matter. I replied I had said something that upset her. "Is it around your name being on the stone? I can see why you would not want to look at your name every time you see the stone. I've designed my burial place and my name is not going on until I die."

"Frank, what do people do when one spouse dies at a relatively young age and the other person remarries? Where does one get buried?"

"It's funny you should mention that," said Frank. "A good friend of mine lived just around the corner. His wife died and he buried her. After a few years he remarried and his second wife died. Fortunately he was able to purchase a third grave right next to the first two. So he buried her and left space for himself in the middle. However, most of the time you're buried with your first love."

Anniversaries too take on added significance after the death of a dearly beloved. Of all the milestones, the anniversary of the day of that person's death will probably be a major event in your life for years to come. Like a few inches of snow on top of a few inches of snow, on top of yet more snow, the cumulative effect can be overwhelming.

Margaux and I started talking about the first anniversary of Nancy's death a month in advance. Whereas I wanted to be in some distant place, Margaux wanted to spend the day at the cemetery. My situation was complicated by the fact that our wedding anniversary occurred two weeks before her death. After much deliberation, we agreed to be sidetracked by Lorna and her daughter, Michelle, the weekend of the wedding anniversary, by being taken on a tour of Niagara Falls.

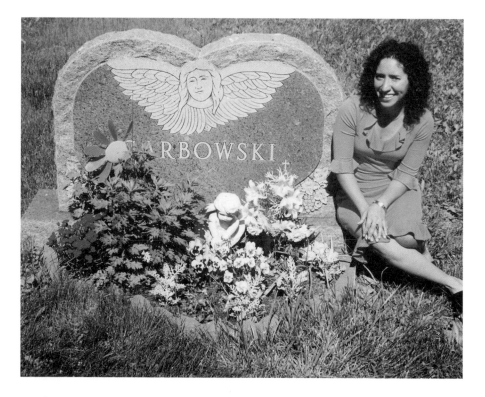

Where the outlines of the stone simulated the wings of an angel, Margaux drew a unique, yet simple shape; an angel's face turned to the side . . . Grape vines were also sketched along both sides near the bottom of the stone, representing one of my passions.

We also agreed to be home and spend time at the cemetery on the day of her death.

About a week before the fateful day, we started discussing what it would feel like, if just the two of us were at the cemetery grieving and it occurred to us that perhaps friends and neighbors would be interested in also attending. At one point we even discussed erecting a tent alongside the grave. Finally, we decided to call a select but inclusive group of friends and neighbors, inviting them to a five o'clock church service on that memorable Saturday. After church we would go over to the cemetery to pray and talk to Nancy. Everyone was then invited to the house for pizza, wine and beer and dessert.

For the first few anniversaries of Nancy's death, the day of the week rather than the exact date remained indelibly marked in my heart. Consequently, on the first anniversary I was emotionally unable to make the transition to the Saturday. I grieved on the Friday.

Margaux had the last day of her summer job that Friday. When I awoke, I felt it was a significant day. I therefore went to the florist, selected a white rose and placed it in a holder with water. While placing the rose on Nancy's grave, I felt very close, as I relived the last few minutes of her sojourn on earth. In real time, I had not been allowed to do that. I wept and wept but little by little I felt better about being there. I remembered how, the first few times after her death, when I brought her flowers, I felt numbed by the fact she could no longer hold them. Nor could she delight in their bright colors or enjoy their lovely fragrance. A year later it felt different. A little better. The white rose now symbolized my eternal love. It was a sign of my being there.

As I stood at the grave, first crying, then thinking about her, I noticed two white butterflies fluttering around. They disappeared as soon as I noticed them, but then, awhile later, they reappeared in the nearby tall grass. I was reminded of Nancy's butterfly phase, of how much butterflies comforted her because they were free to fly about. I recalled her chagrin over the dead butterfly and how she then moved on to the angel phase. It was fitting to see these butterflies just as the foundation was to be dug for Nancy's angel-shaped memorial stone.

By one o'clock on that Friday, my grieving was under control. Once again, Margaux and I were at different places. As was the pattern that summer, she would be grieving on her time schedule the next day. This time discrepancy seemed inevitable and I accepted it as well as I could.

That Saturday was devoted to a rapid yet systemic cleaning of a house that had not received much attention the previous weeks. During this hectic activity, two instances struck me as bizarre and unexplainable. Vacuuming in my bedroom, I lifted the ruffle on my side of the bed and discovered a bright pink turban Nancy had often worn after she lost her hair to chemotherapy. Although I readily admitted to being the world's worst housekeeper, I had recently vacuumed and tidied under the bed. There was therefore no way to explain the presence of this turban except for possibly one incident. Just a day or two earlier, Margaux and I had moved a huge box of pictures from under the other side of the bed. Perhaps, unknowingly, we had dislodged Nancy's turban from a deeper spot. In disbelief, I carefully cleaned off the dust balls and shoved it inside Nancy's dresser drawer.

The previous Wednesday or Thursday I had somehow gotten a nasty grease stain on the tan shorts I was wearing, so I had pulled out a pair of blue shorts I had not worn in awhile. That Saturday morning, feeling a paper in the right pocket, I pulled it out and unfolded a bill from the Jolly Hotel on the Via Veneto in Rome. Nancy and I had stayed there when we enjoyed what was to be her last European trip and her first visit to the village of Alfadena. The Jolly had been the high-point of our trip and by far the finest hotel we had stayed in since the Bauer Grunwald in Venice. It now occurred to me, these two objects simultaneously symbolized the worst horrors and greatest highs we had experienced together. I felt Nancy was hovering nearby. I felt she wanted me to remember the good times as well as the bad. Twenty loving caring friends came to the church service. After the service there was some milling about and conversation. One couple came to the church but could not handle the cemetery. Another person could not handle the service but came to the cemetery and the house.

The cemetery was small and friendly with markers, monuments and plantings of all sorts. Lorna had carefully planned and planted Nancy's favorite colorful flowers in preparation for this sharing moment. The group meandered in slowly, deep in thought. After thanking everyone for coming, I led the group in prayer. Margaux's and my intention was to conduct a candlelight ceremony, centering around the special Padua Italy candle that Nancy and I had, without fail, lit and prayed before, every evening of her last two weeks on earth. Accordingly, at the memorial ceremony, we passed around a white taper to each person. I also wanted to light the Padua candle and pass the flame around the circle. However the spot where Nancy was buried always had a breeze and this day the wind was so strong that no one could keep their candle lit. Without fail however, the flickering flames and Nancy's presence, touched each person's soul.

After saying a few words about Nancy, I encouraged anyone who wanted to share a thought or recollection, to do so with the group. I emphasized that no one should feel obliged to speak. About a third of those present had something to say. When I felt no one was being cut off, I concluded: "Margaux, Lorna and I thank each and every one of you for coming. Now I want to thank you on behalf of Nancy. She always loved people and I know she is happily looking down to see all of us here visiting with her at this time." I rushed the last few words as my emotions welled up and almost prevented me from saying what I wanted.

It was a warm afternoon and back at the house everyone decided to sit on the patio to enjoy the cool breezes coming in from the west. At one point, I missed Margaux and went through the house looking for her. I found her in my bedroom going through the nightstand drawer where Nancy had kept personal cards and journals. She was crying uncontrollably. At last she was connecting with her grieving. I gave her a hug and found a box of tissue for her. I sat there and consoled her. From time to time we would discuss something she found, causing renewed tears. Several times she said she was sorry to be crying. I told her "Let it rip, let it go, cry it out."

While hugging her tightly, I couldn't help but silently recall my own memories concerning Nancy's nightstand drawer. As opposed to people who die suddenly and unexpectedly, many cancer patients have time to prepare for death. This manifests itself in a variety of ways. About three months after Nancy died, I had noticed an envelope in her nightstand. It contained a series of photographs. As I looked at them, they took me back to when she was a child, an adolescent, a bridesmaid and finally a single person in an apartment on New York's Upper East Side. I saw childhood photos of her brother and sister, father and step-mother and various aunts and uncles. Most of those people were now dead.

I remembered asking Nancy about this envelope of photos earlier in the year. At that time, she went to great lengths to frame cabinet photos of her mother and father, which were later prominently displayed near her casket when she was laid out. Nancy told me she was going through pictures to find good ones suitable for framing. I remembered observing that we already had a lot of photos and that wall/display space was at a premium. While she may have intended to frame more of these photographs, it occurred to me she had selected a series of photos capturing only her youth.

Upon more careful analysis and reflection, the photos really were about her progression as a young adult to the

132

point she met me. Our daughter and I were in none of these photos. The series ended with her New York apartment. There were no photos of us after our marriage, even though we lived in that apartment for several years. There was, however, the photograph of her graduation. She was clearly very proud and very happy on that occasion. There were also several photos of her being a bridesmaid and photos of the fateful trip to New York which eventually caused the decision to move to the Big Apple. Little did she know she was destined to meet her husband-to-be several years later, in this Manhattan setting.

There were also snap shots of her apartment on New York's fashionable East Side in her genuine Emilio Pucci blouse which contained all of her favorite colors. I remembered her wearing that blouse on a date with tight black bell bottom pants. Clearly, she had taken time to go back and reflect upon the milestones in her life up to when she had met me.

I found these photographs extremely painful. It hurt to see how she prepared for death while I was in denial of the fact that she would die. I had a twinge of regret that I was unable to go through these photos with her, to ask her what each one meant to her. This was and still is an extension of my hurt and pain over never seeing her again, never hearing her voice again and never hugging her again. What a lost opportunity!

Years after Nancy's death, Margaux, too, would discover there were more than photographs in this nightstand drawer. She came to view this drawer as a sort of journal, documenting what Nancy had to relive in order to prepare herself for death: a lock of hair from Margaux's first haircut, love poems from me, the hospital bracelet she wore when Margaux was born.

Now, here were Margaux and I, that afternoon, huddled together in front of Nancy's precious dresser drawer. I remained objective and supportive to Margaux for as long as she needed me, as I knew that Lorna was hosting the get-together on our behalf during our prolonged absence. In time, Margaux and I went back to sip wine with the remaining friends.

While grieving, I also now understand that one of the more difficult tasks is cleaning out the effects of the dearly departed. In my case, our modest home offered limited closet and storage space. Yet, I just could not muster the initiative to really clean out.   Lorna suggested I box everything and put off going through it until some future time. Damp basement conditions and a sizzling attic in the summer precluded this option—at least that is what I told myself. However, time and time again I would come across something which could trigger intense sadness, grieving and almost depression.   For example, after moving some boxes in the closet, I found a pair of bedroom slippers Nancy had bought for me weeks before she died, with the obvious intention of giving them to me for Christmas. Then there was the box of lovely stationery I had helped her pick out at the mall for Margaux. I mentioned it to Margaux and she could not even look at it.

However, as Lorna pointed out to me, these intended gifts can represent many golden opportunities for the future. While Margaux could not look at the stationery that first Christmas, perhaps by the next Christmas or some future holiday, it would mean a lot to her. In time, she would be receiving something her mother picked out thoughtfully and lovingly with her own hands, when exhaustion made walking from the car to a mall entrance a major challenge.

With the first anniversary of Nancy's death and Margaux's return to school, it was difficult to fully comprehend how Margaux felt. She had been depressed. An image came to mind which helped me understand. I had heard of a Dr. Ballard who utilized amazing technological advances to locate and film the wreck of the Titanic deep down on the ocean floor. The barnacle encrusted hull loomed tall and majestic over the exploratory submarine. Similarly, Nancy's shadow was looming over Margaux, sad, quiet and intimidating.

These modern day explorers identified porcelain dolls, wine bottles and other memorabilia along miles of ocean bottom. Margaux and I were also sifting through remains and memories, each triggering a stream of recollections.

Shortly after this, when my new job did not work out, with Lorna's help, I pursued my dream of starting my own business. However, it backfired as I was not at full strength. Grieving was sapping my energy. The same was true for Margaux. She struggled to focus on her school work. Days of sadness, grieving and melancholy took their toll on both of us.

Close to sixteen months after Nancy died I came to a profound realization. One of my closest friends was right. Life after Nancy's death was hell. 'Being alone' was taking on a new meaning for me. It now involved a struggle I was having with myself and myself alone. Nancy made no further demands on me. Margaux was at school and I thought about her all the time, yet, her education was assured and I was there to help her in any way she required. So, what was troubling me? It was the processing of MY loss and MY pain and MY emptiness and MY anger and MY everything else. Nancy was out of it. I was struggling with myself and it was me and my struggle that was keeping me from feeling good and living life to its fullest.

Then I received a long distance phone call from my cousin Stephen who had previously lost his father in a plane crash. The ten year memorial celebration involved a picnic at the site of the crash. He said this was the first year he did not cry but rather rejoiced in the new friendships he had finally learned to enjoy.

It also takes courage to step out into the world and risk loving another person. It's a tremendous adjustment to suddenly be a single person again. Some single people never heal. Some die of a broken heart. Others remain stuck in a hurt place, unwilling, disinterested or unable to move on to a new life. They also, if there are children involved, immediately enter the ranks of single parenthood, which represents a monumental challenge in its own right.

Even when enough healing has occurred and the survivor is ready to engage in a social life, his/her children may complicate these new friendships as there can be differing points of view concerning a suitable period of mourning. Whereas, a parent might want to go out dancing, a child often wants to be the apple of the parent's eye. Children in general, involved in intense grieving, find it difficult to cope with a parent who has paid their dues and wants to move on and explore new options. Then too, the new person in a single parent's life may not be concerned about how the children feel about them which further complicates their moving on.

Another important aspect of grieving and moving on in life was letting go of a tendency to idolize Nancy. In time I learned to accept Nancy's shortcomings and limitations as well as her strengths, without thinking less of her as a person. We are all human and to do any less would be to grieve and mourn a person who never existed the way we remember them. This balance is also critical to a healthy moving forward, being in touch with reality and being open to new relationships and personalities which like Nancy's, I could not expect to be perfect.

As a middle-aged single, I encountered a lot of caution, pain, hurt and reluctance to engage in new relationships. Some people were just not ready. Others could not get over the fear of being hurt again. Indeed, nature seemed turned inside out and in turmoil.

Now, here's what you can do.....

* Remember, grieving is a very personal, individual experience. There is no grieving timeline as you lose your loved one bit by bit, not all at once.
* Try and face your pain, rather than ignoring or suppressing it.
* At all times, you should do what is right and most comfortable for you.
* Write to, phone or email friends and family as the spirit moves you, going out of your way to be in touch on a somewhat regular basis.
* Push yourself to be sociable. Walk over to a neighbor's house and engage in a conversation.
* Determine what's best for you. Some will gain strength by reaching out to others going through the same experience or about to lose a loved one. However, depending on your personality it may be awhile before you can connect in this special way.

CHAPTER 10
La Vita Nuova — New Life

"Most people are like a falling leaf that drifts and turns in the air, flutters, and falls to the ground. But a few others are like stars which travel one defined path: no wind reaches them, they have within themselves their guide and path."
Siddharta by Hermann Hesse

Until I met Lorna, I was just like that falling leaf. As a youth I had the vision and passion to be a college professor. I was attracted by the prospect of publishing or perishing. However, circumstances in life led me to a career in business that spanned twenty-five years. I was blessed with much success.

In mid-life I gradually came to realize I was not following my star. I began to understand why; for the last twelve years, I had had this gnawing feeling of not belonging.

When Nancy died, the falling leaf of my life no longer drifted and fluttered. It was swept up in a hurricane, a tornado, a storm. I did not know what was happening. My life was spinning violently out of control.

Then, four months later, I met Lorna, who gave me the special gift of letting me search for my inner force. With her infinite wisdom and patience, she guided me, hugged me and helped me heal. She also always encouraged me to pursue my innermost dreams.

I'm getting ahead of myself. Here's how it all began.

Feeling very alone in the empty house, the first December after Nancy died, I pushed myself out to a single parents' dance at a Polish-American club, in a nearby town. En route, I drove through an old section of town that I had never seen before. Many of the buildings were sagging and in disrepair. It was a dark, cold night and this seemed to accentuate the dismal surroundings. I held my breath driving over an old rusting bridge to get to the hall.

Inside, a large number of regular singles were clustered around a long bar which dominated one side of the dimly lit room. There was a tiny dance floor at the back where a disc jockey spun an unending series of uninspired selections. Like a London fog, the acrid smell of smoke penetrated every nook and cranny. To the left there were tables and a small number of singles. I recognized several of them from previous events.

As more singles dribbled in, suddenly a radiant angel entered the room and penetrated the fog. Everyone in the room was blinded and, for me, it was a near-mystical experience. I sauntered up to her and said, "Yo toots, what's a gal like YOU doing in a dump like this?"

"Well, sir, I don't think I really have to tell you as I don't even know your name," the radiant angel replied. Then, inexplicably, she went on, "To tell you the truth, I'm Santa's helper tonight. Look at me as kind of an elf. I'm delivering Christmas gifts for needy children and if everyone else is like you, I'm owtta here!"

Getting back to reality, Lorna was really, initially, at the club to meet a charity representative and drop off her wrapped Christmas gifts for needy children. On her way out, however, she was sidetracked by a mutual friend of ours who introduced her to me. She was tall and slender with long dark hair, reminding me of a sixties' flower child. She had the most engaging smile and her laugh exuded joy and merriment.

We danced a few, but mostly we just talked. The first time we got up to dance, Lorna asked me to hold her car keys as she did not have a purse or pocket.

The group seemed content to leave us alone except for Max, who came over, introduced himself, grabbed a chair and interjected himself between us. He angled his chair away from me, looked directly at Lorna and said, "I've been told you're new to the singles' scene. At this point in your life, you may be vulnerable. Some men are like wolves, out there to take advantage of unsuspecting women like you. Why, I've even heard of men trying to take a woman home the first night they meet."

I felt he was directing his comments at me and I was insulted. At one point, the DJ played a slow song and I whisked Lorna off to the dance floor. I held her tight, but not too tight. Her long shapely body seemed comfortable next to mine. I shared with her both my discomfort with Max and the cigarette smoke. It turned out that Lorna too was allergic to smoke. Consequently, regretfully, neither of us would be able to stay much longer.

We went back to our table and sure enough, immediately, Max came back to resume his lecture. I cut him off, explaining that I was allergic to tobacco smoke and had to leave. He said, "Fine, no problem," and without missing a beat, turned to continue his conversation with Lorna. It was as if he were delighted to see me leave. I purposely interrupted him again saying, "Oh, by the way Lorna, here's your car key. I almost forgot and left with it in my pocket."

Max looked like a boulder had fallen on his head. His jaw sagged in disbelief. I could see he was thinking that perhaps I was a wolf, adept at pocketing a single gal's car key after just a few moments of conversation. As I got into my car, I had to smile, but then I had an uneasy feeling. Perhaps Max was the wolf, disguising himself in a mantle of helpfulness.

Driving home, reflecting on the evening, I felt there was something special about Lorna. She seemed to take a sincere interest in me and how I felt. I was very comfortable talking with her. It turned out that she, too, had been involved in several long lasting caretaking experiences. It seemed like ages since I had experienced the warmth and support of such a genuine, caring presence. I called her the next day and she agreed to meet me for a hamburger at my favorite diner.

From there on, our friendship became extremely complex. Lorna completely threw herself into helping me market my first book. She also took a special interest in my detailed written account of Nancy's personal battle against breast cancer, and suggested that I go a giant step further, and, page by page, express not only Nancy's, but also my innermost feelings during our sixteen year battle. It took years of patience and perseverance on Lorna's part and endless hours of collaboration to give birth to this unique exploration of the male perspective during and after a prolonged battle with a chronic illness, which we fondly christened, "Don't Walk Through The Mirror."

Over and over again, Lorna pointed out, that what I later remembered as happy times, were without fail for her, always punctuated with my memories, thoughts and feelings of active grieving. By sticking with me through these times, Lorna gave me a gift of tremendous magnitude. It was not until years later that I comprehended the depth of my hurt. It was as if Nancy had sent a beautiful, loving, human angel to help me through these seemingly endless difficult times and keep me from breaking.

Lorna also had a unique sidetracking ability. Consequently, what stands out first and foremost during an important business trip we took to Montreal, Canada, were the French restaurants, *le festival du homard*, and a personally guided tour, by Aileen and Murray Shaw of the city, the farmers' market, and the Canadian artists' section of the Museum. However, in reality, our main mission was to promote my first book, which we achieved by working hard and scheduling numerous appointments during which we met with several book distributors, bookstore owners and publishers. Thankfully, the owner of a major chain of Canadian bookstores shared information with us that was to provide tremendous impetus to the marketing effort of my book back in the States.

While in Montreal, I also had the distinct pleasure of meeting Lorna's uncle, Robert Shaw and Johann Shaw, the Deputy Commissioner and First Lady of Expo '67. Decades later they retain legendary status in Canada. Much to my amazement, upon reading my first book, he pointed out how it echoed the very same management principles that made Expo such a success. In his honor, my book was placed in the prestigious McGill Faculty library.

Then too, just two and a half months after we met, my birthday rolled around, and Lorna, sensing my social isolation, engineered a massive surprise party. Somehow she did the detective work to search out and contact my innermost circle of friends, people she did not even know. About two weeks before my actual birthday, we were to go to an Italian restaurant in South Philly with two fun loving friends of mine, Anita and Eddie. Unknown to me, Lorna had made them part of this ploy.

Lorna insisted that the four of us have appetizers at her home before venturing into the city. When my friends and I arrived, Lorna asked me to get a fourth chair from another room. I innocently opened the door and imagine my surprise when I peered into the darkness and suddenly spied a room full of people. When they cried out "Happy Birthday!", all color drained from my face and I instantly staggered backwards. There was genuine overall concern that I might pass out. Scared by my reaction, Lorna even held off taking a photograph. That was a major indicator of just how bad I must have looked, as she was an avid photographer.

It took me a while to overcome the initial shock. This was my first surprise birthday party ever. Not only had I always opposed them, but this one came at the most unexpected time.

Another element of the surprise which caught me completely off-guard, was a carefully timed phone call from my daughter in London. It was great to talk with her at the exact time my friends were celebrating my birthday with me in such a grand style. To this day, I still don't know just how Lorna was able to pull this off.

When I did compose myself, I had a great time. I was amazed how much Lorna thought of me to do something special like this. It was a good feeling to see my best friends gathered together, representing different phases of my life. Some of them had never met before. Above all, it was an uplifting feeling to once again socialize with many of my friends, who, seven months after Nancy's death, still, for varying reasons, had not felt comfortable including me, now a single person, in various activities. Somehow Lorna had taken the pressure off everyone and created a marvelous, relaxed opportunity to congregate and celebrate.

In time I realized that my relationships with married friends would change in response to my new, forced and unwanted marital status. For example, one couple stopped celebrating certain holidays with me, thus canceling out a comforting tradition which had spanned over a decade. At first, I blamed myself and wondered over and over again, what I had done wrong. Finally, after sharing my feelings with them, I discovered that they found it too painful to be with me as it made them miss Nancy even more.

Other dear old friends resented my socializing, my feeble attempt to move forward with my life. Over time, this severely affected several close friendships as I could not help but resent their resentment. How could they possibly know what I was going through? My couple friends were lucky. They still had each other.

Happily for me, however, our empathetic friends Anita and Eddie stepped into the breach and made it a priority for Margaux and I to spend Thanksgiving with them. Consequently, they went out of their way to replace an old pattern with a positive new one, regardless of how much they missed Nancy's presence.

Nothing came naturally any more. While Margaux was studying in London, I planned a vacation with her to Italy during her Spring break. However, as the time approached, I became increasingly aware that this desirable European vacation might disrupt my overall well being. By touring abroad I would be breaking the important grounding process which Lorna had so carefully initiated. How would I get through two weeks without her support and guidance, without even talking on the phone?

I had a delightful vacation with my daughter but once back in the real world, sure enough, I had to reground myself. Lorna quickly pointed out that my daughter and I were on two entirely different healing schedules. Whereas Margaux was postponing true mourning of her mother's death until her return to the States, I had already, before my trip to Europe, begun processing the gut wrenching realization that Nancy was gone forever and had begun dealing with the endless mental and social consequences of her death.

My processing continued during my first solo Easter without Nancy as Margaux was still in London. Once again, Lorna stepped in and with the help of her daughter, Michelle, and Joe Greenstein, I celebrated, rather than suffering through the spring holiday. With their contagious enthusiasm and support, I regained some much needed strength, cutting a huge lilac bouquet from my garden for the Church, and coloring eggs with Lorna. I also brought a special Easter cake for Lorna's home cooked feast. I therefore received much love that first Easter after Nancy's death, yet I also greatly missed her presence. Nevertheless, by introducing Nancy's and my traditional Easter cake to Lorna's present day feast, I had attempted to both comfort myself with the past and celebrate in the moment.

Lorna's daughter, Michelle, was also an important force in my healing. She too offered me precious, unconditional love. As a university student, she presented me with my first computer in an attempt to help me with my home business and later, after I rejoined the corporate work force, Michelle helped set up my company laptop and rescued me when the hard drive crashed. I had a need for her enthusiastic, unconditional love. I had a need to be rescued.

We also enjoyed numerous serious theological debates and deep discussions about the meaning of life. Talking with Michelle took me back to my college days which was a good thing as she was able to pull me back in time, up and over my deep hurt, way back to a happy time. Both

144

Michelle and her special friend, Joe, were always there when I needed them.

Lorna also had an intense contagious passion for Niagara Falls. I had been there twice before and my recollections were extremely indifferent. However, touring the falls with Lorna changed my perspective. Now I love the falls and it will always be a special, beautiful, quiet, get-away place in a hectic world. Looking at photos of Lorna at the falls, her face is the perfect expression of happiness, peace and tranquility. With her, I too, was deeply impressed by both the powerful beauty and the peacefulness of this natural wonder.

Guided by Lorna, I witnessed a place, above the falls, on the Canadian side that I had never before seen. At this special spot, I was right at the edge of the falls, where the water rushed out over the cliff, dashing out into a huge massive free-fall, and then crashing at the bottom of the horseshoe.

Over time, Niagara Falls has consequently come to represent the powerful, tumbling, headlong rush of life. When Nancy died, life did not slow the slightest beat. It maintained its relentless forward momentum. I slowed and stumbled, even stopped at times, yet, life surged on. Picking up the pieces of my life and getting back into the vital flow has been and always will be my personal challenge.

Speaking of personal challenges, Lorna was right, Margaux postponed her grieving when she went back to university right after the funeral. She further delayed grieving when she went to study in Europe for a semester. Consequently, when twenty-one year old Margaux came home from abroad the next summer, we were indeed, in very different places emotionally and mentally.

The very moment she returned, she started active grieving. I too was still grieving, but the important difference was that I had processed a lot during her absence. Margaux's grieving therefore immediately started pulling me backwards, erasing much of the painstaking progress I had made with Lorna's help.

Then too, Lorna quickly sensed Margaux's innocent ambivalence towards her. She explained to me that Margaux would find it very challenging to accept the first caring female person in my life after Nancy. As Lorna was determined to protect our father-daughter relationship, she therefore made the conscious decision to support me emotionally from a distance, so I in turn could support and nurture my daughter. Selflessly, she was preparing the way, so hopefully, Margaux could more easily accept the next important person in my life.

When Lorna started distancing herself, my stomach would turn. Both Lorna and I knew that Margaux was the most important person in my life. In turn, we both knew Margaux was not doing anything intentionally. However, I could not help but resent the fact she was affecting the supportive, loving friendship I was so fortunate to have found. Then too, I also wanted to be a great father. Over the years, Margaux and I had established a very good relationship but when she came home from London, our relationship was weak.

That first summer, I therefore learned what it really meant to be a single parent and it was a real shock to my system. Margaux was a young adult and I was totally unprepared for the amount of parenting she would require. During some intense father-daughter discussions, Margaux explained that she was defending her mother. She felt she was holding the fort alone, even though it felt stupid and futile. Margaux also felt that if she moved along in the grieving process, memories of her mother would be lost forever. She felt moving forward was a threat to her mother's memory.

Ironically, most often, when I was with Lorna, we were deeply engrossed in writing a book in Margaux's mother's memory. It was arduous work and I required all the help, feedback and support Lorna could muster. I also needed Lorna's constant encouragement. However, there was no way Margaux could understand this supportive relationship.

Margaux's and my predicament therefore required a lot of open communication, love and trust between us. Hard work came into play too but, most of all, Margaux and I needed time. As I had no previous experience in such sensitive single parent situations, I needed constant help and advice from an outside source and Lorna cheerfully and quietly provided that much needed support.

In time, Margaux and I took our father-daughter relationship to a new level. When Nancy was alive, while raising Margaux, Nancy had been the enforcer and I was the peacemaker. However, after Nancy's death, I quickly discovered I could not be both father and mother to her. I, too, felt that no one could ever replace her mother. It would never be the way it was, as I had to step up and be the enforcer at times, a role that was totally foreign to me. Thus, with time, my relationship with Margaux changed and evolved. We became closer, discussing and working our way through difficult situations in Margaux's challenging young-adult life. Literally days before she was to return to school, we were thankfully able to come to closure over several major issues.

When Margaux returned to the university, Lorna continued making important contributions to this book. As I previously mentioned, in the original version of "Don't Walk Through the Mirror", I, with the help of Lorna, focused solely on Nancy's emotions and feelings involved with her battle with breast cancer. However, once we completed this version, Lorna insisted we rewrite the book. One by one, she had me match each of Nancy's emotions and feelings with how I felt at that exact moment in time and how I coped during each and every stage of the lengthy battle. Consequently we literally spent thousands of hours probing, discussing and recording my very personal and emotional memories. Lorna also contributed insights into the newest version of the book, based on her ongoing personal experiences from assisting several loved ones through chronic and unfortunately, fatal illnesses. All the while she also took on the complicated task of focusing on my immediate feelings and needs.

Then too, as a single parent, she continued to grapple with overwhelming familial concerns of her own. Meanwhile, I became more and more consumed with writing this book, and believed it to be a manifestation of my over-riding desire to be published. Lorna, however, knew it was, initially, and is, to this day, a very important part of my healing.

As I continued active grieving, I often did not realize all the opportunities I had to support Lorna. Somehow, I was unable to do so. However, Lorna reinforced that this was not a bad thing; it was the way it was. She constantly reminded me that it was unusual to not have any family in the area to help me and Margaux with the grieving process. Lorna had therefore made a conscious decision to try and fill in this void for me, and indirectly, for Margaux, asking me, to quietly, in turn, use the strength she gave me, to support Margaux.

When I finally realized what was happening between us, I was both hurt and confused by the realization that I could not do more. I had given to Nancy for so long, I was unaccustomed to being on the receiving end, with no questions asked. At that time, I had no way of knowing I was totally underestimating the profound extent of my hurt and pain. I was trying to move forward with my life when I was not ready to advance. I needed more time to heal. I needed the new Anthony to come out and take form in the crucible of the world.

On several occasions, I tried to move our unique friendship to a more permanent place but Lorna stated over and over again that it was not right and she pulled back. I did not understand her reaction at the time. However, I now realize that it was fortunate that one of us was able to step back, look ahead, and be objective about my complicated healing process and my daughter's and my bonding after Nancy's death.

All through this, Lorna was there for me: helping with

the manuscript, setting up a fax machine, lining up support when computer problems arose and constantly providing a steady stream of bright, colorful flowers to encourage me to be positive and upbeat. Most importantly, Lorna was always reminding me of how far I had come and how well I was doing. Often I could not see it by myself. Even several years after Nancy's death, I was overwhelmed by the huge empty spot in the middle of my life. At such times I discounted the progress I had made and despaired of ever getting my life on an even keel. It was hard, without Lorna's insight, to recognize that the empty spot, while it would never go away completely, was very slowly diminishing in size. In actual fact, I was ever so slowly gathering strength while defining myself.

At one point in time, both Lorna and I re-entered the singles' world. This time round, I found the dances too crowded, noisy and smoky. The discussion groups were intellectual pabulum, often frequented by individuals with emotional baggage. Whereas the ostensible purpose was to meet eligible bachelors, some women were blatantly bashing men at singles' functions. Lorna, too, came to new realizations. She learned most middle-aged men expected physical closeness, if not intimacy, after the second or third date. This was not in line with her personal values and she did not want to lead anyone on. Thus returning to the singles scene was difficult and confusing for her too.

I found it hard to let go of what our friendship could have become. Just as the tall, full, late-August tomato plant, laden with big ripe fruit represents a dramatic change from the puny seedling planted in the spring, our relationship too, had evolved. However, clinging to the realization that there would always be something unique between us, we then made an important conscious decision to be soul-siblings. As an only child, I began to feel what it was like to have a sister. Not a sister I fought with, but a very special person with whom I could talk and share my hopes and dreams, no matter where life

149

took me.

How well I remember one particular spring Saturday. It was a bright sunny spring day with lilacs, azaleas and dogwood blossoming in splendid color. Driving to a local automobile club, I experienced an astonishing sensation of coming out of a long dark tunnel into the light. This light did not hurt my eyes. At this exact moment, it was as if my eyes had acquired the ability to open wider and draw in more energy; I felt as if I had been in a cave for twenty-two months, hurting, licking my wounds and mourning my loss. In this deep dark recess, I had been preoccupied, futilely trying to recapture what I had lost. I was resisting change; trying to go back; refusing to acknowledge where I was and not going forward. At last, I too, finally understood why Lorna felt my attempts to move to a more permanent relationship would not work.

Peace and calm flowed over me. My eyes were taking in more and more of the light of this beautiful day and all was bright around me. I had a vibrant sensation that I had entered a new phase of my life. It was as if a vital part of me had been in a hospital or a sanitarium for a very long period of time and finally I had been released.

Perhaps this is how Nancy felt when she prepared herself to accept death. She had to let go of the past and step boldly into the future. She seemingly did it peacefully and with tranquility.

Reveling in this moment, I drove to Lorna's house to drop off the maps I had picked up for her at the automobile club. I shared with her the special feelings I was experiencing. We hugged and cried together. Tears of happiness. Mine, for having finally made the next independent step. Lorna cried because she was happy for me. She loved me so much. She had worked so diligently to nurture and support me for over eighteen long difficult months, to bring this light into my life. The joy of that enlightening moment was so intense. However, sadly, I would later learn that this moment was fleeting. My process of moving forward was to ebb and flow like the oceanic tides and Lorna would continue to be there for me.

Although Lorna was now preparing for a long distance trip to care for her ailing father, she assured me that, even though she would be hundreds of miles away for the next few months, she would be next to me in spirit and would keep in touch with me on a daily basis by phone. Her departure brought to mind a poem about God. A person is walking along the seashore and the imprint of God's footsteps appear alongside in the sand. Then the footsteps disappear. The person despairs that God has abandoned them, when in reality, He was carrying them. So it felt with Lorna. I asked myself, must I too journey on my own for awhile to discover my new self?

Part of the answer to this question revealed itself about three and a half years after Nancy's death. I went on a business trip to West Palm Beach, Florida where one of our team-building activities was a deep sea fishing trip. It was a clear warm sunny day in late March. The water was calm and the cooler was full of beer.

Even though I had been fishing since I was seven or eight years old, I had never fished off the Florida coast. I was amazed to learn the Gulf Stream was no more than three miles off shore and that we would be fishing in 250 to 300 feet of water. The Captain fired up the twin screw engines and headed for a wreck. On the way out to sea, I noticed one rod was significantly larger than the others. I fingered the thick line and said to the mate, "What's this, about a hundred pound test?"

"Uh huh," he replied. "And that's a one pound sinker." As he lifted a hatch and netted a live two-pound fish to bait the hook, he explained that the currents were very strong. He then heaved the fish and the sinker over the side as we skirted alongside the wreck.

In just a minute or two, he pulled the rod up, and reeled hurriedly. He hooked a fish and turned to our group for someone to reel it in. First, I was amazed at how quickly and skillfully he had set the hook. I'd fished in deep water off wrecks before and this fellow was incredibly good. Once the fish was safely in the holding tank under the deck, the captain circled around to take another pass alongside the wreck.

Having observed an employee from Malaysia was not feeling well, I encouraged her to go for the next fish. I hoped that getting involved would be the best thing for her. She fought a good sized fish and the mate helped her reel it in by donning thick gloves and pulling up on the line for her. In effect, he helped each individual reel in their fish, while keeping constant pressure on the line to minimize losing it. She landed a 35 pound amberjack.

We made another pass and the other woman in our party landed a good sized barracuda. Now I knew it would be my turn. I did not like someone else hooking my fish, but there was nothing I could do.

When my turn came, I sat in the big chair and as I took the large rod from the mate I said, "If you don't mind, I would rather you not touch the line unless I ask you to." The mate gave me a hard stare but said nothing. I started reeling and lost a fish after just a minute or two. We made another pass at the wreck, the mate hooked another fish and I reeled up, finally noticing the fish jumping out of the water about 30-40 feet away from the boat. It was about a 12-pound bluefish.

"Isn't it strange hooking a bluefish 300 feet down off a wreck?" I asked the mate.

"It sure is. I don't know if I've ever seen one hooked that far down before."

Just then, the fish leaped again and was able to dislodge the hook. Two for two. I lost two fish in a row.

We passed the wreck a third time and the mate quickly hooked another. I started reeling and the line quickly went limp. When I reeled up, we could see the line had been bitten off.

"Sharks. Has to be sharks or blue fish down there," said the mate as he swiftly and skillfully created a wire leader. Meanwhile, the captain roared off towards another wreck.

It was still my turn. I had lost three fish. During the

first pass along the new wreck, the mate hooked a fish and handed me the rod. Feeling the vigorous, heavy pull on the line, I knew this was a big fish.

"Reel up fast!" cried the captain from up above. "You have to get that fish out of the shark zone right away or you'll lose it!"

I was reeling as hard and as fast as I could. The fish was coming up steadily. Just when I estimated I was in the clear, it felt as if a huge hand had grabbed the line. It was tight and taut and try as hard as I could, I could not get the reel to turn. In fact, the line started going out a bit.

"A shark's got your fish!" cried the mate excitedly.

All of a sudden, the hand released and I started reeling in feverishly. The line was coming up.

"There's still something on the line," I hollered.

"The shark ate half your fish," stated the mate.

Reaching into my years of fishing experience, I kept reeling as fast as I could, vigorously pulling the rod high up in the air to give my half-fish the illusion of motion as the shark watched it continue to ascend. Suddenly the huge pull returned. The reel stopped in spite of my efforts. Slowly, silently, the tip of the rod started to dip relentlessly towards the water.

"Now you have the shark! You've hooked the shark!" exclaimed the mate.

I held on, feeling the power of the fish.

I had asked the mate not to touch my line. He had honored my request, yet, he was good enough to instruct when I should pull up steadily on the rod. Furthermore, he told me when to wait at the top of the arc and then let the rod down, reeling as hard and fast as I could and when to pull the rod up again. Waiting, then reeling.

Every now and then there would be a stalemate. The fish would resist and I could not reel. I observed the back of the boat being pulled down towards the water, the ocean splashing onto the deck.

At other times, the fish would head for the bottom and the line would zing off the reel. In these runs the fish was taking back feet of line that I had so painstakingly achieved.

Once, the big shark was so powerfully insistent, I could feel my body being pulled out of the seat.

The mate then tried to help me by putting a harness around my lower back and hooking it to both sides of the reel. The idea was to let my body do some of the work. With the harness, I noticed that when I reeled down, I could only go halfway due to the shooting pain in my lower back. "This will not work," I thought to myself. I tried it a few more times and finally decided I could not take a chance on hurting my back, which had already been compromised. I called out to my boss, Rodney, and asked him if he would like to take a turn. He eagerly came forward. I abandoned the seat, the mate secured the back harness on my boss and the fight resumed.

Now the mate played a major role with his gloved hands, skillfully helping bring the fish closer to the surface. At one point, we could see it under the water alongside the boat.

"It's about a 450 pounder!" roared the captain. He called to me and said, "That shark head would make a great trophy in your living room. That's a great head mount. We can do it for you for about seven hundred dollars."

"How do we get the fish in the boat?" I asked, suddenly realizing that no one was going to be able to haul that fish into the boat alive.

"I'll shoot it with a shot gun, then we pull it in through that lower hatch over there," replied the captain.

The fish was so close to the surface, the mate was able to retrieve his sinker and some of the tackle.

Just then, the fish flexed its great power and headed for the bottom with the line singing off the reel. We took another ten minutes or so to bring the fish up near the surface again. One of our party tried, unsuccessfully, to take a photograph. No sooner did the fish approach the boat when it suddenly pulled down and away.

"What do you say? It's a great head mount. Huge

shark. 450-pounder," boomed the captain.

"Nah, I'm not interested. Let it go," I said. The mate cut the fish loose and we raced back to the dock.

Back on shore, I was in a contemplative mood. I was glad the fish did not have to be shot. I felt humble after the experience, but I was also upset I had nothing to show. I knew if I talked about it, people would immediately chalk it up to a fisherman's tale. So, I remained silent, electing not to talk about it at all.

From all this I came to understand eternity exists only in the present. The past does not exist. If only we could let go of it. The only part of the past which should be brought forward are all the positive, loving joyful experiences. Since no one can predict the future, ultimately we should all try to live fully in the present, which is, of course, more easily said than done.

I finally realized that this had been my dilemma ever since Nancy had died. I had been living in the past, missing her, feeling this huge empty spot in the middle of my life, feeling sorry for myself. Then I looked at relationships and became frustrated when they would not promise to develop into the future relationships I desired, nor the past relationship I missed so dearly. All through this, I was not living fully in the present.

Similarly, the reality of my fight with the great shark was in the present. I had to let go of expectations and concepts of how I had learned to fish in the past. It was best to let the fish live rather than make a trophy of it, in effect, trying to drag the past into the future.

The next day of the business meeting we had a half-day stress reduction session with a ninth degree Black Belt. Frank had had a near-death experience several years ago. During his recovery he had to learn anew how to talk, tie his shoes and do many other things we take for granted every day. His goal in his new life was to use meditation techniques to help terminally ill patients. He wanted to give them an alternative, or an adjunct therapy, to traditional surgery and chemotherapy. All afternoon I could feel energy pulsing back and forth between us, clear across the room.

Frank sat on the floor in front of us and talked about his efforts to attain the coveted tenth degree Black Belt. He sought out individuals who had accomplished that achievement, asking them what they did and how they did it. He then went off and did everything suggested by those accomplished individuals. He explained to us that it was as if the tenth degree were on the carpet right there in front of him. As he consciously reached out to grasp it, it would move away and elude him, no matter what he did. I recalled the night after Nancy had died, recording the musical tape for the funeral viewing. I had felt Nancy right there next to me. When I reached out to hug her, the feeling disappeared.

Frank also talked about his vision of helping the terminally ill with breathing and meditation. He had prepared a comprehensive presentation. He made lists and called on every health care provider in his community, presenting his outstanding new concept, which could be used in conjunction with traditional treatments. While there was interest, there were no takers.

Obsessed with his need to be in a position where he could make a difference in people's lives, Frank pitched his ideas to people he met at parties, in food stores, anywhere and everywhere. Whenever he met someone in the health care field, he tried to win them over.

After months of exhausting, focused, concentrated effort, Frank stepped back to observe what was going on. He finally saw a similarity between obtaining the 10th degree Black Belt and selling his concept. Tired and discouraged, he decided to let it go. He would devote his energies to something else for a while. If it was meant to happen, it would have happened.

The next day he was invited to a cocktail party. He went and enjoyed a relaxing evening, meeting all sorts of people, making polite yet interesting social conversation. The very next morning Frank's phone rang. It was the Director of a major health care provider whom he had met the previous evening. He was impressed with Frank's mastery of oriental breathing and meditation techniques. This Director had an idea that Frank's approach just might be very beneficial to the terminally-ill patients in his facility. He asked if Frank would be interested in putting his techniques into action.

The afternoon of our business meeting, Frank led us in an awareness and awakening exercise that involved breathing. We all relaxed in our chairs, closed our eyes and were instructed to keep our mind from wandering, to think of our breathing and nothing else. Frank turned on a tape machine and the sound of oriental wind instruments filled the room. Then he instructed us to "Breathe in the new. Hold the breath to absorb the energy. Breathe out the old. Relax. Sink into the surface supporting you. Let go." Frank repeated this exercise with minor variations for a half hour. At the end of the session, he walked around the room and gave each and every one of us tapes to take home.

For months afterwards, I would set aside ten to fifteen minutes each morning to do my breathing and deep relaxation exercises. I played Frank's meditation tape on the clock-radio-tape player that Lorna had given me as a Christmas gift. Wanting to personalize the gift, Lorna had attached a plaque with the inscription: "Wishing you many happy awakenings." When presented with the gift, I remember Lorna's asking me if "awakening" was a word. I assured her it was. After many months of playing Frank's tape, one morning I happened to look at the plastic tape holder and finally noticed that the title of his tape was also, "Awakenings." Indeed, living the life of a single person had, and would continue to be a process of gradual "awakenings".

On the tape I could hear birds chirping, water gurgling and oriental wind instruments in the background. Side one of the tape was an elementary version of the awakening exercise. Side two was an advanced class. While concentrating on breathing and listening to side two of the tape, I looked straight ahead at nothing in particular, and extended my hands to the side, slowly bringing the tips of my index fingers together. Not moving my eyes, not even looking directly at my fingers, I then slowly moved my hands apart and to the side. Amazingly, as my fingers separated, I thought I saw a white light where they had been; a white light which connected them even though they were physically apart. In the moment I did not understand what that meant. Now I believe in the energy of the life force which is inside each and every one of us. Under special circumstances, our inner energy can be seen as a light. Like the white light between my fingers, it's always moving from living object to living object.

While death is an inseparable part of living, the energy itself never dies, it is always dynamic. For example, observe the lowly rock. On the surface it appears to be inert, yet, like me, its atoms and molecules pulse with the same vital energy. Then too, water is incessantly vital and changing. It evaporates, forming clouds high in the sky. It then falls to earth as rain and with its incredible tensile strength, it can flow from the highest peaks, down to the deepest valleys, down to the depths of the ocean floor.

At times, while meditating, I sense that I am one with this life force and that I am one with plants, especially succulent plants, without the benefit of a woody skeleton. See how they wilt and droop when they need water, when their life energy ebbs. How fragile and vulnerable they are.

I am also one with the animals, birds and fish who have the same life blood pulsing through their veins, fighting, living and loving as we do. During such moments I am indeed one with the universe.

Amazingly, after the West Palm Beach trip, the emptiness in the middle of my life was, once again, temporarily gone. In the moment, I realized I did not need another person to make me happy and complete in the present. In the moment, all I needed to do was to live fully in the present, making the most of each precious moment.

At this point in time, I had also changed my approach to life substantially.

Slowly, imperceptibly at first, I had changed from being a driven, type "A" personality, and thus I was, no longer, always aggressively pursuing very structured goals. Lorna had been the primary force behind this profound change, patiently teaching me to relax more and get in touch with my inner impulses and to empathize. Other life experiences reinforced this new outlook on life. When in doubt, or when faced with a difficult decision, I now turn inside myself, alert to subtle nuances in and around me, indicating the correct path to take.

I am so fortunate. I have a beautiful, intelligent, loving daughter; a wonderful human being whom Nancy and I brought into this world. She will continue to make Nancy and me proud in the coming years and I will always treasure time spent with her. I have my health, my house, a track record of success in business and a rapidly growing list of publications. Furthermore, I've gained a sister soul mate with whom I will always be able to share my innermost feelings.

I can't help but wonder how many people never recover from a loss such as mine. How many of them could discover a meaningful new life if they had help, as I did, along the way?

I close my eyes and I see that tiny Polish hall and the tall slender smiling gal with the long dark hair. Tears of gratitude pour down my face.

I close my eyes and I see a little girl at the Trevi fountain, clutching a pink fuzzy animal. The smile on her face denotes a simple joy, traveling with her mom and dad.

I close my eyes and I see a young woman in her twenties in form-fitting jeans and a tight top. In my mind's eye, I am young and we are picnicking in Central Park. There is no photograph of this magical moment in a courtship that led to a long and happy marriage.

Memories of the past, an abundance of blessings in the present and the exciting potential of a new life.....this is where I am now and I am grateful for this wonderful opportunity.

The falling leaf, swirling in the storm, has been transformed into a blinking star. At this moment, it appears stationary in the sky. It's too early to tell if it will soar or fall to the earth and crash. Chances are, it's imperceptibly moving in the right direction.

TO EACH HIS OWN

Nurture strength of spirit to shield you in sudden misfortune.

Do not distress yourself with dark imaginings.
Many fears are born of fatigue and loneliness.

Whatever your labours and aspirations, in the noisy confusion of life, keep peace in your soul.
With all its sham, drudgery and broken dreams,
it still is a beautiful world.

Beyond a wholesome discipline, be gentle with yourself.
You are a child of the universe no less than the trees and the stars; you have a right to be here.
And whether it is clear or not to you, no doubt the universe is unfolding as it should.

Be cheerful.

STRIVE TO BE HAPPY!

(Quoted from Desiderata, author unknown)

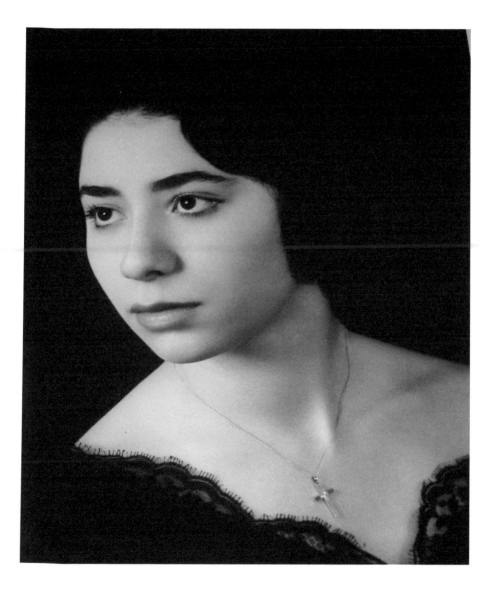